MEDICAL ETHICS SERIES

David H. Smith and Robert M. Veatch, Editors

The Search for an

▲
───────────────────────────────────
▼

AIDS VACCINE

*Ethical Issues in
the Development and
Testing of a Preventive
HIV Vaccine*

Christine Grady, R.N., Ph.D.

Indiana University Press

BLOOMINGTON AND INDIANAPOLIS

© 1995 by Christine Grady

The paper used in this publication meets the minimum requirements of
American National Standard for Information Sciences—Permanence of
Paper for Printed Library Materials, ANSI Z39.48-1984.

MANUFACTURED IN THE UNITED STATES OF AMERICA

Library of Congress Cataloging–in–Publication Data

Grady, Christine.
    The search for an AIDS vaccine : ethical issues in the development
and testing of a preventive HIV vaccine / Christine Grady.
        p.   cm. — (Medical ethics series)
    Includes bibliographical references and index.
    ISBN 0-253-32619-2
    1. AIDS (Disease)—Vaccination—Moral and ethical aspects.
2. AIDS (Disease)—Prevention—Moral and ethical aspects.   3. AIDS
(Disease)—Research—Moral and ethical aspects.   4. Clinical trials—
Moral and ethical aspects.   I. Title.   II. Series.
RA644.A25G73   1995
174' .2—dc20   94-35650

1 2 3 4 5 00 99 98 97 96 95

Contents

▲
▼

Dedication and Acknowledgments

▼

This work is dedicated to my family, who have supported me with love and understanding throughout this endeavor; and especially to my patients, who have taught me so much about courage and perseverance.

I am extremely grateful for the responsiveness and assistance of many individuals who provided me with information, helpful discussions, thoughtful guidance, and encouragement. In particular I would like to thank:

- Leroy Walters, Ph.D., my mentor
- Alisa Carse, Ph.D., and John Fletcher, Ph.D., my dissertation committee
- Maurice Hilleman, Ph.D.
- Jack Killen, M.D., and many others at the Division of AIDS, NIAID, especially the Vaccine Branch
- John LaMontagne, Ph.D., and others at the Division of Microbiology and Infectious Diseases, NIAID
- Robert Chanock, M.D.
- Joan Porter, Ph.D.
- Mary Ropka, Ph.D., and others at the Clinical Therapeutics Laboratory, NINR
- Glenna Jo Oliver

THE SEARCH FOR AN AIDS VACCINE

INTRODUCTION

▲
_____
▼

> HIV vaccine trials will . . . be among the greatest public
> health research challenges faced to date. (Vermund,
> p. 13)

> We must develop ethical and legal answers that are as
> sophisticated as the science that develops the vaccine
> itself. (Charles McCarthy, as quoted by Weisburd,
> p. 329)

Developing a vaccine to prevent infection
with the human immunodeficiency virus (HIV) is a global priority because
of the enormous public health need and the lack of alternative methods of
prevention adequate to achieve control. Development of any vaccine requires
careful, systematic testing from the level of basic science through definitive
testing in human beings. The goal of this book is to examine the ethical challenges inherent in the development and testing of a preventive vaccine
against HIV and to suggest strategies for meeting them. Ethical challenges
include the justification for doing the necessary human-subjects research in
the search for a vaccine as well as the particulars of how the research should
be done.

THE MAGNITUDE OF THE HIV PROBLEM

HIV infection is a rapidly spreading global
epidemic with staggering human, economic, and social costs. By 1992, the
World Health Organization (WHO) reported that at least 10 million adults
had been infected with HIV (Mann).[1] WHO estimates that at least 20 million adults and 10 million children will become infected during the 1990s (a
cumulative 40 million or more by the turn of the century), with the largest
proportional growth occurring in Asia, Latin America, and Africa. In the
United States, an estimated 1 million people are infected with HIV, and more
than 400,000 have been reported as having acquired immunodeficiency syndrome (AIDS).

But the large and growing numbers of infected persons are only part of the story. Most of those who become infected with HIV develop symptomatic disease, AIDS, within ten to fifteen years. AIDS is a devastating multisystem disease accompanied by significant morbidity and disability and a high fatality rate. By 1995 the cumulative global number of adults with AIDS is expected to increase from greater than 1 million today to approximately 4 million (Mann, p. 246). HIV will result in the deaths of more than 75 percent of those infected (Francis, p. 1444)—in reality, probably 100 percent with time. One writer predicted that the AIDS epidemic could, "before its end, fell one quarter of the globe's population" (Gould, p. 33).

Added to the high fatality rate and the long incubation period is the fact that the majority of persons with AIDS are young adults. AIDS and HIV disease were found to be the leading cause of death for men ages 25 to 44 in sixty-four American cities in 1990 (and the second leading cause of death in the same group nationwide), and the number one cause of death for women ages 25 to 44 in nine cities in five states (Selik, Chu, and Buehler). Estimates of years of potential life lost due to AIDS are between 1.2 and 1.4 million for 1991 (ranking it third among all diseases in the U.S.) and 1.5 and 2.1 million for 1992. AIDS will clearly outstrip all other diseases in lost human potential (Federal Coordinating Committee on Science, Engineering, and Technology [FCCSET]). Children are the group with the fastest rate of new infections.

The costs of caring for people with AIDS and HIV disease are enormous. "Assuming an average (U.S.) of $100,000 for direct medical costs of each AIDS case, the costs of the epidemic are immense ($75 billion for infections to date, plus $3–6 billion for new infections occurring each year)" (Francis, p. 1444). In addition, caring for people sick with AIDS is complex and labor-intensive, and the problem is complicated by inadequate health care delivery and limited (and expensive) treatment options. Three antiretroviral drugs (zidovudine, dideoxyinosine, and dideoxycytidine), all with the ability to stall the progression of HIV-related symptoms, have been approved in the U.S. The usefulness of these drugs has been hampered by toxicity, the development of resistance, controversy over their long-term effect, and cost. Antiretroviral treatment is not likely to be able to control the epidemic anywhere, especially not in developing countries or inner cities, where treatment is often unavailable.

AIDS orphans are another tragic manifestation of the HIV pandemic. WHO estimates that by the year 2000, in addition to the 10 million HIV-infected children, another 10 million will be orphans because of AIDS (International Council of Nursing [ICN], p. 1). "Unless the course of the epidemic changes dramatically, the overall number of motherless children and adolescents (in the U.S.) by the year 2000 will exceed 80,000 . . . [with] the vast majority . . . from poor communities of color" (Michaels and Levine, p. 3456). In Uganda alone, about 1 million children were estimated in 1991 to be AIDS orphans (ICN). The problems caused by children orphaned because of AIDS are "so large and complex in nature that existing facilities, infrastructures, resources . . . are presently not enough" (National Council for International Health, as quoted by ICN, p. 1).

"From whatever perspective—number of HIV infected people, number of people with AIDS, number of AIDS orphans, or the stresses on health systems and entire societies," it is clear that the future will be worse than the past (Mann, p. 246). The ever-increasing numbers of persons infected, sick, or dying from HIV have an obvious impact on society in the U.S. and the world. The epidemic has also been associated with major social disruption and social changes, which are perhaps less obvious and certainly less well understood. Increasingly a disease of the "underclass" (Bayer, 1991), HIV/AIDS will affect and be affected by the culture and politics that surround those who are at greatest risk.

> HIV has demonstrated its ability to spread across all social, cultural, economic, and political borders. It is now clear that HIV will eventually reach most, if not all, human communities and that while geography may delay exposure to the pandemic, it will not ultimately protect any community. (Mann, p. 246)

SOCIAL AND POLITICAL ATTITUDES TOWARD THE PROBLEM

There is a curious popular tendency to believe that the danger from HIV has peaked and is declining as a result of information and education programs. This view is seriously flawed, for today global vulnerability to HIV is increasing in response to social, economic, and political events (Mann), and the incidence of infection continues to rise unabated. Similarly, there is an ever-present sentiment that HIV is associated with social deviance, and therefore it is someone else's ("their") disease and problem. Unfortunately, this sentiment has been reinforced recently in the U.S. by the changing demographics of HIV disease and by reports (and distorted media interpretation of same) such as the recent *The Social Impact of AIDS in the United States* by the National Research Council (1993). The National Research Council cautions that because HIV is endemic in already deprived and segregated populations, this attitude may only increase and HIV/AIDS will "disappear, not because, like smallpox, it has been eliminated, but because those who continue to be affected by it are socially invisible, beyond the sight and attention of the majority population" (NRC, p. 9).

Since the beginning of the epidemic in the U.S., there have been complaints from numerous sources that the public and private response to the problem has been too slow and inadequate. The Presidential Commission on the HIV Epidemic, the National Commission on AIDS, and panels at the Institute of Medicine, among others, have claimed that the federal response was woefully inadequate and that there has been an absence of leadership in a clear crisis. Lack of leadership, lack of adequate attention and resources, and bureaucratic intransigence have all been publicly criticized by AIDS activists. In the last couple of years, this sentiment has been countered by "a growing public sentiment that AIDS has received more than its share of media attention, resources, and social indulgence" (Murphy, p. 7). This backlash criticizing the effort and resources that have been devoted to HIV, coupled with a sense of HIV being a problem of social deviance, continues to threaten the adequacy of efforts to control the epidemic.

NEED FOR CONTROL
OF THE HIV EPIDEMIC

"A vaccine is urgently needed for control of global disease" (FCCSET, p. 3). Because of the magnitude of the problem, there is a humanitarian need to find reliable means of prevention, control, and/or treatment of HIV infection and disease. Current preventive measures hold little hope for adequately controlling the spread of HIV. Nor will control be achievable with current treatments, which are toxic, not curative, and not universally available. Reliable means of prevention, control, or treatment will be found only through carefully done research. "We have, in the international as well as the national sense of 'public,' a vital public health interest in stopping it [HIV]. By extension of this logic, we have a vital public health interest in protecting, and possibly enhancing, the power of the single most important weapon we bring to the battle—our ability to make scientific medical progress" (Dixon, p. 122). In addition to a vital public health interest, it has been asserted that there is a general ethical responsibility to do research on treatment and prevention: "Those who fund research (national and international, public and private) have an ethical responsibility to employ research as one means of improving medical care and protecting the health of the people" (Council for International Organizations of Medical Sciences [CIOMS], 1992, p. 4).

PREVENTION THROUGH VACCINATION

Given the number of people with HIV infection, increasing health care needs and costs, the absence of effective means of prevention or treatment, and the increasing prevalence of AIDS among socially "powerless" people, it is critical that a vaccine be developed. AIDS is and has been a top public health priority of the U.S. government, and the creation of a preventive vaccine has been one of the chief objectives (for example, see U.S. Public Health Service [USPHS], 1988, p. 54). Developing an effective HIV vaccine is also an international priority of the WHO.

Control of Viral Infections through Vaccines
Vaccines are generally safe, effective, and inexpensive ways to control diseases, including many viral infections. For example, measles is controlled in most parts of the world, poliomyelitis has essentially been eliminated from the Americas, and smallpox was eradicated from the world, all through vac-

cines (FCCSET, p. 26). Nonetheless, there has been limited success in the development of vaccines against retroviral infections (HIV is a retrovirus), and against sexually transmitted diseases (HIV is an STD). HIV behaves very differently from most other vaccine-preventable viral diseases, so developing an effective vaccine is a complex task. Despite these differences and the impressive scientific obstacles faced to date (see chapter 4), most involved scientists believe that the development of an anti-HIV vaccine is possible.

The Inadequacy of Current HIV Prevention Methods
Current prevention activities throughout the world focus on identifying and modifying behaviors that put people at risk for acquiring HIV infection. While such information, education, and counseling are important, they are not sufficient to curb the global HIV epidemic (FCCSET, p. 26). The effectiveness of preventive efforts depends to a great extent on individual motivation and on particular circumstances. Additionally, many of these methods have not been proven successful. Prevention of infection is believed possible for the autonomous individual willing to take certain steps to avoid exposure.[2] It could be accomplished most of the time by shunning risk behaviors (abstaining from sex with infected partners or partners with unknown infection status; avoiding the use of needles or unclean needles; not working with blood), and less consistently by using available means of reducing risk (e.g., condoms, clean needles, fewer sexual partners). Behaviors which put one at risk of HIV, however, are mostly private behaviors and can be notoriously difficult to change because they are "linked to deep biological and psychological drives and desires" (Bayer, p. 11). Increased knowledge about risk does not necessarily lead to a change in behavior. Additionally and importantly, some people are at risk not because of voluntary behaviors but for other reasons (e.g., neonates born to infected mothers, recipients of infected blood products, victims of sexual violence). Since current preventive efforts offer little hope of curbing the rapid spread of HIV, many believe the only way to control the epidemic is through an effective vaccine.

Risk behaviors which lead to infection, although private and difficult to change, are associated with serious social consequences. "Our collective fate is utterly dependent upon private choices, choices made in the most intimate of settings beyond the observation of even the most thoroughgoing surveillance" (Bayer, p. 11). Thus an effective vaccine to prevent HIV is a highly desirable social priority. Without one, we are dependent on a sense of constraint and individual responsibility which will shape intimate choices and behaviors. Evidence to date suggests that this will be insufficient to control HIV. "Like all grave social challenges, the AIDS epidemic thus imposes the necessity of transcending the self-interested perspective so characteristic of everyday life. It demands the emergence of a sense of communal responsibility" (ibid., pp. 11–12). Perhaps capturing and nurturing some of this emerging communal responsibility would facilitate the development of a vaccine which, if effective, could allow for more choices and less need for constraint at the level of personal behavior. In addition, a vaccine might enable people at risk for HIV to live more normal lives; "the only hope for enabling that to occur and for significantly arresting the alarming spread of the virus is the development of an effective vaccine" (Gostin, 1987, p. 9).

THE COMPLEXITY OF VACCINE DEVELOPMENT

Vaccine development and evaluation involve basic research, preclinical evaluation and production, and clinical trials with human subjects. Proving the efficacy of any vaccine is a lengthy, complex, and expensive task, and companies that invest money in research and development want to not only recoup their losses but also make a profit. In the 1980s, the expected average cost of development of any vaccine was estimated at between $20 and $30 million (IOM/NAS, 1985b, p. 45). Clinical trials of HIV vaccines will need to be very large and very long, and therefore more costly, in order to answer questions of efficacy.[3]

The ideal HIV vaccine should be safe enough to administer to large numbers of healthy adults and children; able to elicit protective immune responses (which will probably include humoral, cell-mediated, and mucosal) in a very high proportion of vaccinees; able to protect against various strains of virus or at least locally relevant strains; able to induce long lasting protection with a minimal number of doses or boosters (since many at risk for HIV infection have poor access to health care, long duration of protection is particularly desirable); easy to administer (orally would be best); heat-stable, sterile, and easy to transport to remote geographic areas without cold storage or sterilization facilities; and inexpensive, especially since HIV is primarily a problem of underdeveloped countries and people of low socioeconomic status. While many scientists believe the development of such a vaccine is possible, others are more skeptical.

OBSTACLES TO VACCINE DEVELOPMENT

Although the worldwide effort to develop a safe and effective vaccine against HIV is unprecedented in modern science, it has faced formidable challenges and has been hampered by the diversity and complexity of viral antigens, a lack of understanding of the immune response to the virus, the lack of an adequate animal model, and the long incubation period between infection and symptoms of disease, among others. Because of the enormity and urgency of the public health need, clinical trials of vaccine candidates in human subjects are ongoing while intensive basic and preclinical research continues. Gaps in current knowledge will most likely be filled through further evaluation of vaccines in human clinical trials. Evidence from animal studies now shows that protection is possible,[4] and Phase I and II clinical trials conducted to date have shown some preventive HIV vaccine candidates to be safe and immunogenic. What remains to be shown is whether induced immune responses in vaccinated humans can be protective against infection or disease.

Successful development and evaluation of an effective HIV vaccine will require a large and continued commitment. Critical elements include:
—Additional scientific knowledge relevant to the virus and its interaction with its human host;
—Close collaboration among governments, scientists, and manufacturers in vaccine development;
—Attention to ethical, legal, and social considerations. (FCCSET, p. 5)

Complete evaluation of promising vaccine candidates will require national and international field trials, each of which will be long and costly and involve thousands of volunteers. No HIV vaccine candidate is yet ready for field trials of efficacy. However, it is not only the science which is not ready for the task; a number of ethical, political, and social issues must be resolved before such trials should be started. At the same time, the social and political pressures to find a vaccine soon are enormous. It has even been predicted that the earlier use of a less effective HIV vaccine will prevent more infections than waiting for a more effective one.[5]

Using syphilis as the paradigm, Brandt speculates that the development of effective treatments and vaccines will not immediately or easily end the epidemic because HIV is a sexually transmitted disease and one accompanied by fear, hostilities, and intolerance of social deviance (1988, p. 367). He warns that it is highly unlikely that a sufficient number of people will identify themselves as at risk and utilize the vaccine, at least initially. Others have argued against focusing scientific efforts and resources on a vaccine to prevent HIV infection because it can be prevented by avoiding certain high-risk behaviors. However, as mentioned above, many people at risk from HIV do not accept risk voluntarily, and even those who engage in high-risk behaviors do not always do so fully voluntarily. In addition, for some, being able to engage in sexual activity and bear (healthy) children will be possible only with an effective vaccine.

There are also possible risks to society associated with having an effective vaccine against HIV. Since the efficacy of any vaccine is likely to be less than 100 percent, reliance on a vaccine for protection may influence some persons to employ other means of protection from infection less often or less consistently. Practicing more risk behavior rather than less could limit the impact of an effective vaccine on reducing the incidence of HIV infection and disease. Also, the existence of a moderately effective vaccine could make future testing of other, possibly more effective vaccines much more difficult and less of a priority. Directing resources toward the creation of an HIV vaccine also diverts them away from developing treatment for HIV disease or other diseases. None of these arguments presents a good reason not to pursue the production of an HIV vaccine. The development of a safe and effective vaccine against this virus is an urgent social good and priority, with potentially great benefits for the global society.

The risks of *not* pursuing research to develop and test an HIV vaccine include increased global incidence, morbidity, and mortality from HIV disease, with continued tragic human and economic consequences. Unless and until there is an effective and widely utilized means of preventing and treating HIV disease, it will continue to devastate many of the world's peoples, and particularly the poorest nations of the world. In the U.S., the epidemic is "settling into spatially and socially isolated groups . . . concentrating in pools of persons who are also caught in a 'synergism of plagues': poverty, poor health and lack of health care, inadequate education, joblessness, hopelessness, and social disintegration [which] converge to ravage personal and social life . . . [and] foster and aggravate HIV infection and AIDS" (NRC, p. 7). An effective, widely utilized HIV vaccine could serve to minimize this devastation, and therefore the benefits far outweigh any potential risks.

My interest in this topic stems from several coincidental experiences. First of all, working for the past ten years with HIV-infected persons participating in clinical trials of experimental therapies has made me particularly interested in the ethical justification of human-subjects research and ethical guidance concerning its conduct. Having been fortunate enough to work very closely with research subjects and glimpse some of the hopes and doubts from their perspective, I have gained a better appreciation of the value of well-done clinical research for individuals and society, as well as the strengths and vulnerabilities of those who volunteer to participate. I have been particularly impressed by the influence of political and other nonscientific forces in shaping the HIV research agenda and the conduct of certain research protocols, and by the power of scientific competition.

I have also had the opportunity to participate in implementing the first Phase I trial of a preventive HIV vaccine in the U.S. I was intimately involved in the details of that protocol and deeply concerned about the unknowns and ethical implications. In collaboration with others, I undertook a study to describe the motivations of persons volunteering for this Phase I study (Barrick et al.). Additionally, as a member of the staff of the President's Commission on the HIV Epidemic (1987–88), I began to struggle with the larger, societal and international questions related to prevention and control of HIV infection. The formidable challenges facing the conduct of a Phase I trial of an HIV vaccine were dwarfed by consideration of the future imperatives of testing such vaccines for efficacy. Concurrent with these activities were my studies in philosophy. Thus the seed was planted for this volume.

In considering the challenges of developing and testing an HIV vaccine, I extensively reviewed the relevant literature, including writings on the goals, purposes, and methods of vaccination and the history of the development and testing of many previous vaccines. This history is fascinating and filled with many examples of what by today's standards would be considered ethically suspect or unacceptable. From this review, it became clear that HIV is not an "ordinary" virus, and that developing an effective HIV vaccine may require radical scientific approaches. The scientific possibilities today, which far exceed those of any previous time, make new and radical approaches feasible. Nonetheless, our understanding of the science of vaccines, the best methods for testing them, and the nonscientific forces that influence their development, evaluation, and use come primarily from the rich history of previous vaccines. These experiences, positive and negative, have also helped to shape federal regulations governing the testing and licensing of vaccines, and commercial interest in and willingness to develop vaccines.

Randomized clinical trials (RCTs) with human subjects are the generally accepted method of demonstrating the efficacy of biologicals (such as vaccines) and therapeutics. Discussion of, guidelines for, and controversy over the ethical conduct of RCTs abound. I reviewed available guidance, regulations, and a voluminous body of related literature concerning the conduct of human-subjects research. Again, much of what is the norm today stems from the experiences of the past. The preponderance of current guidance emphasizes the absolute obligation to protect the rights and welfare (and interests) of individual subjects. This obligation is fulfilled through strict adherence to the following points: informed consent from an autonomous adult or an authorized proxy; a favorable risk/benefit ratio for the individual subject; protection of confidentiality; and equity in selection of subjects. The process for ensuring that each research proposal follows these rules is mandatory independent review and approval by an institutional review board. Specific methodological features unique to conducting RCTs, such as randomization and placebo control, have always been controversial, and have been visibly challenged in clinical trials of HIV-related therapies. In chapter 2 I trace the history of guidelines, regulations, and attitudes concerning the ethical conduct of human-subjects research. An important part of this history is the recent changes in attitudes and regulations that have evolved primarily because of the HIV epidemic. Also noted is the apparent lack of recognition of what I find to be salient differences between clinical research on vaccines (and probably other intrusive preventive interventions) and on therapies.

Vaccines result from a synthesis of public health need, scientific possibility, and social acceptability and values (Dull and Bryan, p. 118). The public health need and scientific possibilities for the development of an HIV vaccine are immense. The ethical challenges are enormous and complex. A virtual explosion of contributions concerning the scientific and logistical challenges of HIV vaccine development can be found in the recent scientific literature. Many of these articles mention, discuss, or refer to relevant ethical issues, yet no in-depth analysis of these issues has been undertaken. As difficult as some of the scientific challenges to the development of an HIV vaccine are, ethical questions may constitute a stumbling block equally or perhaps more formidable. Some of these issues are generic to all vaccine research, and some are specific to HIV vaccine research. In chapter 3 I examine the differences between vaccine research and drug research, and the justification for, and current guidance governing, human-subjects research. Reviewing current interpretations of the Belmont principles, the Declaration of Helsinki, and U.S. regulations as a foundation, I examine their adequacy in relation to conducting vaccine clinical trials in general and to HIV specifically. I explore the idea of the community as the primary beneficiary of research. Borrowing from Veatch (1987), I suggest a model of a three-way partnership between investigator, community, and members of the community as the basis for the ethical conduct of vaccine research. I also explore the risks and benefits of the research effort to find an effective vaccine to prevent HIV, including the benefits and risks of having an effective vaccine (the outcome) and the benefits and risks associated with developing and testing potential vaccines (the process).

In chapter 4 I review the current state of the science and the scientific challenges faced in the search for a preventive HIV vaccine. I briefly look at some of the basic and preclinical research, and what has been done thus far in Phase I and II clinical trials. Scientific accomplishments to date as well as social and political influences will help to set the future agenda.

Because Phase I and II clinical trials of preventive HIV vaccines are already ongoing, the next step in the development of an HIV vaccine is the conduct of field trials to determine efficacy. I address issues important to the ethical implementation of Phase III efficacy trials in chapter 5. There I consider the ethical implications of when to start, what the goals are, whom to include, how trials should be designed, how participants' rights should be protected, and what review and approval is necessary. I suggest strategies for Phase III trials that incorporate the concepts proposed in chapter 3.

SCOPE AND LIMITATIONS

The science and politics of HIV are rapidly changing. I have tried to obtain the most up-to-date references, many of which were not yet published, and have attended numerous meetings where these issues were discussed. Also, the people I have spoken with have been enormously helpful in sharing information. Nonetheless, inevitably some of the facts I present will have changed by the time they are put on paper.

There has been enormous recent interest and activity in the field of therapeutic vaccines. I have purposely said little about therapeutic vaccines because I find the ethical issues surrounding their testing materially similar to those of other therapies and different from those of preventive vaccines. I have focused therefore on issues related to the testing of *preventive* HIV vaccines.

Although HIV vaccine efficacy trials will inevitably be conducted in some developing countries, I have dealt only cursorily with issues specific to conducting international trials. My perspective, my resources, and the available literature all argued convincingly for a limited treatment of such issues.

There are bound to be many practical difficulties in selecting communities to participate in vaccine research and in the conduct of "town meetings," community negotiations, and community consent. I am aware of the intense competition in science and the desire to be first to develop an

HIV vaccine. I am also aware that most laypeople do not have a basis for understanding science and the methods of research. Nonetheless, with appropriate attention to explaining the goals, methods, and uncertainties of research, acknowledgment of a common goal to prevent HIV and the role of vaccine research, and empowerment of the members of communities to be "partners" in this endeavor, the necessary research is achievable.

CHAPTER ONE

▲
_____
▼

Vaccines and Their Development: Historical, Social, and Scientific Perspectives

HISTORICAL PERSPECTIVES

Immunization or vaccination is essentially a method of enhancing a person's ability to fight infection. Vaccination is the artificial introduction of any preparation of antigen (e.g., virus, bacteria, parasite, toxin) in a modified form in order to induce a specific immune response to that antigen and thereby prevent or modify infectious disease on subsequent exposure to the corresponding agent. Vaccination against infection is based on the observation that people who have had an infection once are often protected from further infections with the same organism. In most instances immunity is based on induction of antibody or other immunologic responses that persist for long periods of time. "Immunologic memory" allows these experienced immune components to recognize and respond rapidly to an antigen on subsequent exposure, effectively eliminating the antigen. A vaccine is a substance sufficiently like the organism to generate a specific response in the immune system, but sufficiently different that the vaccine does not itself cause the infectious disease.

TYPES OF VACCINES

Vaccines can be divided into two broad categories: live vaccines, which utilize a weakened or attenuated infectious agent to mimic natural infection, and inactivated agents or components of them, which are able neither to replicate nor to infect the host. Each vaccine usually contains, in addition to the desired antigen or its parts, suspension fluids, preservatives, stabilizers, and/or adjuvants. Undesirable reactions can occur not only to the antigen itself but also to these added components and to retained impurities (Grossman and Cohen, p. 724). داداركري(ج)

Live attenuated vaccines induce an immune response most like that resulting from natural infection. Live-virus vaccines, defined by their ability to replicate within the host, are attenuated or weakened with respect to pathogenicity (ability to produce disease), induce cell-mediated immunity in addition to humoral immunity, and usually provide longer-lasting protection than do most killed vaccines (Finn and Plotkin; Hinman, Bart, and Orenstein). However, because they are live and replicating, they are plagued by the ability to revert to a more pathogenic form *in vivo*. They also have retained virulence for at least part of the population, causing reactions, and may in some cases be contagious to those who come in contact with the vaccinee.[6] Live-virus vaccines licensed to date have been made by modification of the virus in cell culture (e.g., measles, mumps, rubella, polio) or by using variants from other species (e.g., smallpox). Scientists are now able to alter the structure of viruses at the molecular level, permitting rational design for attenuation rather than relying on selection of variants by serial passage in animals, *in vitro,* or at altered temperatures (Ellis, 1988, p. 568).

The chances for development of practical attenuated-virus vaccines are increased by the application of viral genetics and DNA sequence analysis. Identified regions in the viral genome can be altered or deleted in order to reduce viral pathogenicity. If more than a single site is mutated, genetically altered viruses are unlikely to revert to more pathogenic forms *in vivo.* Sometimes genetically altered live viruses are used as vectors (carriers) for other viral genes.[7] Genes that code for viral proteins capable of inducing effective immunity are incorporated into the unrelated vector. (Besides viruses such as vaccinia and adenoviruses, bacteria have also been used as vectors.) This technology may allow for single recombinant vaccines that protect against more than one disease at the same time (Ellis, 1988; Plotkin and Plotkin, 1988).

Inactivated vaccines (sometimes referred to as "killed"), on the other hand, do not replicate in the host and are unable to actually infect the host or contacts. They are often less efficient in inducing immunity, so that repeated immunization may be necessary for complete or long-term protection (Finn and Plotkin; Hinman, Bart, and Orenstein). Because of their inability to replicate, killed antigens are given in far larger amounts than is required for live-virus immunogens. Purity is sometimes difficult to achieve, increasing the chances for reactions. Often an adjuvant is used to enhance the immune response. Since they do not replicate, inactivated organisms cannot revert to cause the infectious disease. Classic approaches to making inactivated vaccines have included inactivating or killing (usually with heat, chemicals, or irradiation) the whole pathogen (e.g., pertussis and influenza vaccines); detoxification of toxoids from bacteria (e.g., diphtheria or tetanus vaccines) by use of formaldehyde; purification of surface components of viruses or bacteria (e.g., pneumococcal polysaccharide or plasma-derived hepatitis B vaccine); and conjugating surface components to other carrier molecules (e.g., *hemophilus influenza b* vaccine) (Ellis, 1988).

Molecular biology has also opened up new avenues for the development of inactivated vaccines. Recombinant DNA technology has been used to mass-produce nonliving antigenic protein components for use as vaccines. Recombinant yeast hepatitis B vaccine, made using antigen produced in a recombinant expression system in yeast, is the first, and to date the only, recombinant DNA (rDNA) vaccine licensed for use in humans. Other methods for preparing nonliving antigens for vaccines being used experimentally include the chemical synthesis of immunogenic peptides, the production of monoclonal anti-idiotypic antibody, and the creation of viruslike particles (Aldovini, Young, and Palker; Ellis, 1988, p. 573).

Vaccines which contain only parts of the organism, rather than the organism itself, are referred to as subunit vaccines, regardless of whether they are made by purifying antigenic components, by recombinant synthesis of proteins, or by chemical synthesis of peptides. In general, subunit vaccines are considered safe, though often not as immunogenic.

GOALS OF VACCINES

The goal of vaccination for the individual is to safely stimulate enough of an immune response that, upon subsequent exposure to that same antigen, the person will remain well or suffer from a milder illness. Stated another way, the goal for the individual is either to prevent infection *or* to prevent clinical disease (i.e., infection is not prevented, but only subclinical infection occurs because of vaccine-induced immunity). A vaccine could also potentially be used "therapeutically," to bolster immunity and prevent progression of disease in someone who is already infected, although this goal has never been successfully accomplished.

Another equally important goal of immunization is the indirect protection of groups or whole populations of individuals; this is referred to as herd immunity. When individuals within a group are immunized, the susceptible host population becomes smaller and the chance of spreading infection to others is reduced or eliminated. (The immunes protect the susceptibles.) Effectively, when a sufficient number of people are immunized, the risk of transmission to an unimmunized person is reduced (Anderson; Fletcher, Fletcher, and Wagner; Finn and Plotkin).[8]

The word *vaccine* was originally coined by Edward Jenner for the material he used to infect persons with cowpox (Latin for "cow" = *vacca*; cowpox is also known as vaccinia) in order to protect them against smallpox. Louis Pasteur broadened the scope of the term by calling his attenuated anthrax cultures used to produce immunity "vaccines" as a tribute to Jenner. Later, suspensions of many other microorganisms or of tissues infected with microorganisms were referred to as vaccines, as were toxins and toxoids. Today, any agent used to induce active immunity (the production of specific antibody and/or cellular responses) is called a vaccine (Grossman and Cohen). For the purposes of this book, *vaccination* and *immunization* will be used interchangeably.

Vaccination as a deliberate attempt to protect people against disease has an interesting and long history. Immunization seems to have been practiced in crude form in antiquity. The oldest recorded form of the artificial induction of immunity is *variolation,* the term given to inoculation with the virus from mild cases of variola or smallpox (Parish, p. 7; Petricciani et al., 1989). There is evidence that the ancient Chinese tried to prevent smallpox with inoculation from as early as the sixth century A.D. (Parish; Plotkin and Plotkin, 1988). Documentation of methods to inoculate against smallpox are found in ninth-century Chinese textbooks (Plotkin and Plotkin, 1988). In China, smallpox was transmitted artificially by blowing the dried scabs from smallpox pustules into the nose. In India, Brahman priests used cotton infected with smallpox "lymph" to inoculate into scratches in the skin. The worship of the smallpox goddess and sprinkling of the site with water from the sacred River Ganges was believed to be an essential part of the success of this practice (Parish, p. 8). The Greeks injected material from smallpox sores in the sign of the cross—the forehead, chest, and both arms (Williams).

The first scientific attempt to control an infectious disease (smallpox) by means of a deliberate systematic inoculation was accomplished by Edward Jenner in the 1790s. Jenner did not know anything about microbes, nor did he understand the mode of action of vaccination; his methods were purely empiric. Because of Jenner's success, in the eighteenth and nineteenth centuries attempts were made in various countries to inoculate human beings or animals with infectious material from other infectious diseases, such as measles, gonorrhea, and syphilis. But the nature of these diseases was unknown, and these attempts were sporadic, tentative, unsuccessful, and often dangerous (Dowling, p. 24). Almost ninety years after Jenner's famous experiment, Louis Pasteur developed a vaccine against rabies for use in human beings. In the interim, scientific knowledge essential ultimately to the development of vaccines was evolving, including bacteriology, mechanisms of infection, and the beginnings of immunology. The concept of contagion was only vaguely appreciated until the work of Pasteur. Robert Koch brought new technology to the study of microbes when he developed methods for isolation and culture. He proved a causal relationship between the anthrax bacillus and disease in 1876 (Parish; Plotkin and Plotkin, 1988) and identified *Vibrio cholerae* as the cause of cholera in 1883 (Plotkin and Plotkin, 1988).

The late 1800s were a very productive time for vaccine development. Pfeiffer and Kolle in Germany and Wright in England developed killed typhoid vaccines (Dowling; Parish; Plotkin and Plotkin, 1988, p. 3). Yersin, Calmette, and Borelli developed a killed animal vaccine against *Pasteurella pestis* (the plague) (Parish; Plotkin and Plotkin, 1985; Plotkin and Plotkin, 1988). W. Haffkine developed a plague vaccine for use in humans, first injected himself, and within weeks had vaccinated 8,000 persons! (Dull and Bryan; Parish; Plotkin and Plotkin, 1985; Plotkin and Plotkin, 1988). Kolle developed a heat-killed cholera vaccine in 1896 (Parish; Plotkin and Plotkin, 1985; Plotkin and Plotkin, 1988). Pasteur, Emil von Behring, Robert Koch, Paul Ehrlich, Elie Metchnikoff, and their contemporaries explored and described fundamental principles of microbiology and immunology which

provided the foundation for much of the subsequent development of biologicals (Dowling; Dull and Bryan; Plotkin and Plotkin, 1985; Plotkin and
Plotkin, 1988). By 1900 there were two virus vaccines, both live: Jenner's
original vaccine against smallpox and Pasteur's rabies vaccine; and three
bacterial vaccines, all killed: against typhoid fever, cholera, and the plague
for use in human beings.

The chemical detoxification of the toxins of diphtheria and tetanus
early in the twentieth century resulted in two highly effective toxoid vaccines
which have virtually eliminated these diseases in much of the world (Plotkin
and Plotkin, 1985, p. 86). The Bacille Calmette-Guerin (BCG) vaccine
against tuberculosis was developed in the early 1920s, but its effectiveness
remains to be proven to the present time. Pertussis vaccine was prepared in
the 1920s from whole killed organisms (ibid., p. 87). By 1935, Max Theiler
had developed a live attenuated vaccine against yellow fever (ibid.). Crude
vaccines were also made from influenza virus (1941) and various rickettsia
(1938), grown and harvested from embryonated hens' eggs (Plotkin and
Plotkin, 1985).

The "golden age" of vaccine development started in 1949 with the
Nobel Prize–winning discovery of John Enders, Tom Weller, and Fred Robbins that virus could be propagated in human cell culture (Beale; Plotkin and
Plotkin, 1988; Robbins, 1977). They were first able to grow Lansing type II
poliovirus in human cell culture (Plotkin and Plotkin, 1988); prior to this
time all viruses were grown in animals or embryonic tissue. The ability to
grow human viruses outside a living host, in a relatively easy and safe
manner, led to an explosion of creative activity in vaccinology. This tech-
nique plus greater knowledge of pathogens and host responses led in the
1950s and 1960s to the development of effective viral vaccines against poliomyelitis, measles, mumps, and rubella (Beale; La Montagne and Curlin;
Plotkin and Plotkin, 1988). The use of vaccines to prevent disease due to
pertussis, diphtheria, tetanus, poliomyelitis, measles, mumps, and rubella
has resulted in massive reductions in the burden of these infections throughout the world (La Montagne and Curlin).

These benefits are unevenly distributed in the world, however. Although
these diseases are preventable by vaccination, there still occur throughout the
world each year approximately a half-million cases of paralytic polio, two
and a half million deaths from measles and its complications, and about two
million deaths from neonatal tetanus and pertussis, all in tiny children, and
most in the developing world (Weisse).

The eradication of smallpox through a global vaccination campaign in
the late 1970s is one of the most important accomplishments of modern
medical science. Poliomyelitis and measles, viral diseases which have caused
significant morbidity and mortality, and for which, like smallpox, the only
reservoir is human beings, have also been targeted as potential candidates
for eradication. In the 1970s and 1980s three effective bacterial vaccines
were developed containing purified capsular polysaccharides: a meningococ-
cal vaccine by Artenstein and colleagues in 1970; a pneumococcal vaccine

by Austrian and colleagues in 1976; and a *Hemophilus influenza* type b vaccine by Anderson and colleagues and Schneerson and colleagues in 1971 and 1972 (Plotkin and Plotkin, 1988). In 1981, a hepatitis B vaccine (Hilleman and colleagues), made from surface antigen derived from human plasma, was licensed, and this was followed in 1986 by a recombinant hepatitis B vaccine, the first of its kind.

The advent of molecular biology and the development of new techniques in genetic manipulation and recombination of DNA (rDNA) have greatly expanded the number of possible approaches for vaccine development. Genes coding for biologically active substances have been identified and analyzed. Techniques for transferring this genetic material within and between organisms with the expression of specific proteins under controlled conditions have been applied to vaccine development (Zuckerman, 1988), allowing for improvement in the manufacturing process and an increased supply of some vaccines. These new techniques have also made possible the development of vaccines that were not possible before.

THE DEVELOPMENT
AND TESTING OF VACCINES

SOCIAL ACCEPTANCE OF VACCINES AND COMMERCIAL INTEREST

> Vaccination is always under attack by civil libertarians who claim the right to be ill, by religious zealots who believe the will of God includes death and disease, and by a legal system that profits from the failure of most people to understand risk-benefit ratios or public health issues. Short memories also ensure that people do not recall the way it was before vaccination. (Plotkin and Mortimer, p. xi)

Vaccination, sanitation practices, and antimicrobials may be the greatest achievements in medicine, responsible for the dramatic lengthening of the average human lifespan, especially in developed countries. Estimates are that the average life expectancy in Roman times was about 22 years, while currently in many of the developed countries of the world it is about 76 years (Hilleman, 1985; Parish). For certain diseases, the impact of effective immunization is most clearly reflected in the decline in incidence of the corresponding disease. For example, in the U.S. there were approximately 206,939 reported cases of diphtheria in 1921 and none in 1986; 21,269 reported cases of paralytic polio in 1952 and only 3 in 1986; and approximately 20,000 cases of congenital rubella in 1964–65 compared to 14 in 1986 (Hinman). Smallpox, a disease which purportedly devastated whole civilizations, was eradicated from the world through vaccination. The prevention of infectious diseases by immunization is generally safe, acceptably reactogenic, relatively simple to deliver, cheap, and extraordinarily effective.

Although the social and economic value of preventing infectious diseases through vaccination is well recognized and the benefit-to-cost ratios

for immunization programs are better than for most other health procedures, "ironically it is at least as or perhaps more difficult to accomplish the
use of vaccines as it is to develop them. . . . It must be remembered that vaccines will only be considered useful if they are used. There is a critical need,
therefore, to perceive the practical while pursuing the possible" (Hilleman,
1985, pp. 416–417). The use of a vaccine is influenced by many factors, including perceived susceptibility to the infectious disease, the real and
perceived benefits and risks of the vaccine itself, the cost of the vaccine, and
the convenience or inconvenience of getting it.

Despite the remarkable achievements of vaccine prophylaxis, the use of
vaccines has always been controversial. The controversy is based primarily
on issues of safety (LaMontagne and Curlin). Some see vaccination as
dangerous and unnatural First, the appropriate population to vaccinate in
order to prevent infectious disease is a healthy population who *might* be at
risk of exposure to the putative agent only at some future time. Sometimes
the most appropriate population to vaccinate in order to control disease by
inducing herd immunity is healthy infants or children, who may constitute
the reservoir for continuing infections with the agent. Vaccination entails
introducing biologic material (such as live virus) that could be harmful into
these healthy persons. No vaccine is completely safe in all recipients, nor is
any completely effective. Some are safer than others, but none that has yet
been used has been entirely free from complications (which range from very
mild to life-threatening) or accidents of one sort or another, although serious
side effects are extremely rare. It is usually impossible to determine whether
there is a causal or only a temporal association between vaccination and a
subsequent adverse event, so the true risk of immunization is hard to calcu-
late. Because of the risks associated with vaccines, standards for safety,
production and testing procedures, and requirements for licensure are
controlled by governmental licensing authorities. In the U.S. this is carried
out by the Center for Biologicals Evaluation and Research (CBER) of the U.S.
Food and Drug Administration (FDA).

For a vaccine to be acceptable to the public despite the potential for
harm, the perceived benefit from the vaccine (even a future benefit) must
clearly outweigh the perceived risk. The perception of the risk-benefit relationship varies with the disease to be prevented and the human needs and
concerns it generates. For example, during the years when poliomyelitis was
epidemic, the risk of developing paralytic poliomyelitis was generally perceived to be high; thus people were more likely to accept some risk
associated with the vaccine in exchange for the protection it provided. On
the other hand, four years after the plasma-derived hepatitis B vaccine had
been licensed, only about 5 percent of the total population and 10 percent
of health care workers at risk had been immunized (Hilleman, 1985,
p. 416). Even health care workers perceived themselves (incorrectly) to be at
low risk of infection and were concerned about a potential risk from the
vaccine (such as contamination with HIV or other viruses), so utilization
was low for several years.

The goal of vaccination is in part to benefit the vaccinated individual (i.e., to protect him/her against infection or disease), in part to benefit others by decreasing the likelihood that they will be exposed (herd immunity, the result of reducing circulation of the infecting agent in the population), and in part to benefit the community at risk and society in general by decreasing the incidence of a given infection and its associated morbidity, mortality, and costs. Because of the benefits that go beyond the individual, and which historically have been enormous, some immunizations have been legally compulsory, and some small risk to the individual has been tolerated. Ultimately, if an infectious disease has been controlled or nearly eliminated, the risks associated with vaccination will exceed those associated with infection. Hence, the balance of interests between the individual (vaccine-associated risks and benefits) and the group (benefits of herd immunity) changes, and interests oftentimes come into conflict (Anderson, p. 932; Fine and Clarkson).

As effective vaccines are used in a community and the incidence of infection and disease drops, so do the actual and perceived risks from the disease. Paradoxically, the acceptability of the vaccine by the public may be affected because as the perceived risk of disease decreases, the perceived risks of vaccination may seem greater.

> Immunization does not capture the imagination as does a new and dramatically successful treatment of a hitherto dire and fatal disease. Immunization is done when a person is well. If a sufficient proportion of susceptibles in a community are protected, the disease decreases, and the previous impact of its morbidity and mortality on the individual and the community are forgotten. Almost inevitably this leads to a slackening in uptake of vaccination and the very real risk of recrudescence of disease. (Cockburn, p. 3)

Fear of side effects may lead to a decrease in vaccine coverage, which in turn may spur public health officials to use a more efficacious vaccine if one is available or can be developed. In some cases, vaccines with greater efficacy have greater complication rates, further increasing the conflict between the individual and the group (Anderson). Inadequate coverage of a population by immunization may also lead to an increase in morbidity and disease in the population (ibid., p. 931).

The phenomenon of complacency about infectious diseases and fear of the possible side effects of vaccines has become a problem in the U.S. in the last twenty to thirty years, and has been compounded by a large number of individual lawsuits claiming vaccine-induced injury or damage. The complacency, due probably to a lack of visibility of vaccine-preventable diseases, was partially overcome by government immunization programs and laws requiring pediatric immunizations before attending school.

Litigation for vaccine-related injuries, however, precipitated a crisis in vaccine supply by the mid-1980s. Much of the fear and the litigation was fueled by adverse publicity in the media. Because some vaccines are required by law, those who believe they have been injured by vaccines feel entitled to compensation.

> Persons who respond to government promotion of or legal requirements for vaccination often benefit others in society, as well as themselves, because of reduced disease transmission. Those who are injured as an unfortunate consequence of immunization should be provided reasonable compensation in a rapid and equitable manner. (IOM/NAS, 1985b, p. 2)

Parents of children who suffered vaccine-related injuries had few options to cope with random tragedy. Health insurance rarely covered their long-term needs; as a result, they resorted to suing the manufacturers for producing defective vaccines or failing to adequately warn them of the risks. A group of parents believing their children to have been injured by the diphtheria-pertussis-tetanus (DPT) vaccine formed a lobby group called Distressed Parents Together. Product liability insurance premiums for manufacturers of vaccines increased dramatically, as did the price of certain vaccines (such as DPT). A reexamination of the economic consequences of the continued production of vaccines resulted in the withdrawal in 1984 of two of three manufacturers of DPT, although the number of domestic producers of all vaccines had been declining since the 1960s (Mariner, 1992b, p. 256).

The U.S. is still heavily dependent on sole suppliers (either manufacturers or distributors), with two commercial companies dominating the market for pediatric vaccines. The litigation claims against the sole remaining distributor of DPT and oral polio vaccines (OPV) were believed to exceed the yearly earnings from the sale of these vaccines in the early 1980s (Peter, p. 981). The result was a shortage of the DPT vaccine in early 1985, and a recommendation from the Centers for Disease Control that the fourth and fifth doses of the vaccine be postponed until supplies returned to normal. Public health officials worried that if manufacturers or distributors abandoned the vaccine market, the country might be left without an adequate domestic supply of vaccine, jeopardizing the public health. Yet, the Institute of Medicine in examining this problem noted that the U.S. had no contingency plan for dealing with a situation in which no commercial manufacturer was willing to produce a major childhood vaccine (IOM/NAS, 1985b).

> Unbelievably, vaccines are under legal attack in the society that has gained the most from their widespread use. Side reactions to vaccines, either real or imagined, are not tolerated, even though they occur at a considerably lower frequency than reactions to drugs. This litigious situation has already had a baleful effect on vaccine manufacturing and is likely to grow worse. (Plotkin and Plotkin, 1985, p. 101)

The process of vaccine development includes basic research, development, testing, production, and marketing, involving numerous organizations in both the public and private sectors. Basic research, needed to identify the pertinent characteristics of the pathogen and the host's immune response, is extremely time-consuming and expensive, and is usually conducted in federally funded academic or government laboratories. Once there is some scientifically promising information, a manufacturer may begin to look at some other factors such as the impact of the infectious disease, the estimated costs of developing, producing, and distributing a vaccine, the ranking of this vaccine against other priorities, and the potential utilization of and market for a vaccine, which is dependent on public acceptance and health care provider enthusiasm. The availability of a vaccine for the public depends entirely on the willingness of a commercial manufacturer to produce it. More than concern about the public health, it is concern about market forces that drives most decisions. "Drug companies are in business to make money. . . . Lots of money in pursuit of more money has a life of its own, if not a mind of its own, and although the agenda of the market is (hopefully) not absolutely inconsistent with the public interest, it would be foolish to look for perfect coincidence" (Dixon, p. 80). Many factors have adversely affected the commercial attractiveness of vaccine development, including the expense and logistics of clinical testing, the comparatively small market compared to drugs,[9] technical problems, liability risks, and a perception that vaccines have received less effective patent protection than drugs (FCCSET; IOM/NAS, 1985b).

If interested, a sponsor or manufacturer must complete extensive, complex work to provide evidence of the safety and efficacy of the vaccine and file an investigational new drug application (IND) with the FDA to do clinical testing in humans. If the vaccine looks marketable after clinical testing is completed, the manufacturer in the U.S. files a license application with CBER/FDA. CBER staff review the documents and convene an advisory committee to provide advice. If satisfied that the product is safe and effective and the directions for use are adequate, the FDA will grant a license. Each vaccine and each manufacturer require a license.

The rising costs of health care and the limited resources available for health care in most of the world mandate rigorous assessment of costs and benefits for all medical interventions. In all analyses to date, effective immunization programs have been shown to be less costly than most other preventive health strategies and far less expensive than the cost of treating established disease (Finn and Plotkin, p. 477). It is estimated that the eradication of smallpox resulted in a savings of approximately $1 billion per year, not including the more substantial savings in terms of the elimination of disease, disability, and death from smallpox. Nonetheless, the costs of developing and testing a vaccine are enormous, as are programs of continuing surveillance. The high costs, coupled with uncertainty about a vaccine's effectiveness and utilization, limited sales potential, a perception of difficulties with patent protection, and the fear of liability, have created a powerful disincentive for pharmaceutical industries to do vaccine research and development.

The necessity for rigorous cost-benefit analysis and the possibility of serious problems in supply resulting from these disincentives for the manufacturers of vaccines led to a series of meetings in the early 1980s to study these issues. Most of these meetings were coordinated by the U.S. Public Health Service or by the National Institute of Allergy and Infectious

Disease (NIAID), the branch of the NIH primarily responsible for vaccine development. Through an NIAID contract, a Committee on Issues and Priorities for New Vaccine Development was established within the Institute of Medicine (IOM) of the National Academy of Sciences to design a coordinated and comprehensive approach to setting priorities for accelerated vaccine development in the U.S., and for international use, especially in developing countries. The committee developed a quantitative model which ranked vaccine candidates according to two main characteristics: (1) expected health benefits, including disease burden from the pathogen, value judgments on the undesirability of conditions arising from the disease, proportion of the disease falling in target groups, various predictions on vaccine development (probability of success) and characteristics (safety and efficacy), likely utilization of the vaccine, and estimated time before the benefits would be achieved; and (2) expected net savings of health resources, including costs of developing the vaccine, the likely cost of the vaccine program, and expected cost savings from treatment and morbidity averted (IOM/NAS, 1985a, 1986).

Using this quantitative model, the IOM committee examined fourteen diseases of importance to the U.S. and nineteen diseases of importance to the developing world for which new or improved vaccine candidates were judged technically feasible within a decade, and recommended a priority scheme. The committee examined costs and benefits from an aggregate societal perspective. It recommended the use of this model for future deliberations about priorities for vaccine development and urged the consideration of nonquantifiable factors (such as administrative, ethical, and political) in making final selections for accelerated development. The committee also said that "final selections . . . and ultimate choices should be addressed in a broader political/public policy forum" (IOM/NAS, 1985a, p. 15). The IOM committee noted that an HIV vaccine was not included in their list of priorities because the state of the science was very young at the time, and the possibility of having a vaccine within ten years was negligible. An important part of the IOM analysis was a projection of the likelihood of utilization of a vaccine by the target population. As of April 1993, the IOM's process had not been repeated, and many of the vaccines that were identified as priorities (especially for developing countries) have not yet been developed because of manufacturer reluctance (Robbins and Freeman).

Concurrently in the mid-1980s, a Committee on Public–Private Sector Relations in Vaccine Innovation was established within the Institute of Medicine to examine and find solutions for concerns about market and liability disincentives for vaccine manufacturers and threats to the public health from a decline in vaccine innovation. The committee's report, "Vaccine Supply and Innovation" (1985b), examined barriers and impediments to vaccine innovation and availability and recommended (1) the creation of a vaccine commission to coordinate, oversee, anticipate, and resolve problems in vaccine development, supply, and use; and (2) the creation of a consistent and just approach to the issues of liability for vaccine-related injury and compensation for those injured.

Several groups studied the options for vaccine injury compensation and protection of manufacturers from liability. Finally, the National Vaccine Injury Compensation Program was passed by Congress in 1986 and became effective in October 1988 (Mariner, 1992b, pp. 256, 261). The legislation included the creation of a National Vaccine Program (NVP) to encourage research to improve the safety of vaccines, require reporting of adverse events, and improve public information on vaccines. The NVP's responsibility is to "coordinate and provide direction for" vaccine research, development, safety and efficacy testing, licensing, production, distribution, and evaluation of the effectiveness and adverse effects of vaccines (Public Law 99–660, Section 2102(a) 1–8). As of April 1993, the NVP still had no consistent operating budget, limited authority, and no approved strategic plan. It has not been involved in coordinating or directing research related to HIV vaccines but has focused primarily on strategies to increase utilization of childhood vaccines.

The same 1986 legislation also established a program to provide no-fault compensation to persons with certain defined injuries from vaccines used to prevent seven childhood diseases. The program was designed to deal with retrospective and prospective cases of injury within specified limits. To date, it has been hampered primarily by insufficient funding and disputes over which injuries should be compensated (Mariner, 1992b, p. 264). One major difficulty has been making causal associations between clinical problems and vaccines.

Liability issues may prove to be especially problematic in the case of an HIV vaccine. Evidence exists that manufacturers' concerns over liability have inhibited or delayed the progress of research in HIV vaccines (NIAID, Overview of AIDS Liability Issues, November 1992). Because the federal government has no legal authority to resolve liability concerns, nor any administrative or contractual resolutions, the only option for liability protection may be legislative. Yet, liability for an HIV vaccine could not be covered under a program such as that described above because the magnitude and probability of legal liability cannot be defined or quantified, and it is not known whether predictable side effects will be delineated. "We cannot talk about legislative liability for a product which is not yet produced or used" (Tim Westmoreland, speaking at the Institute of Medicine Roundtable, December 1992).

DEVELOPMENT AND TESTING OF VACCINES

The progression of a vaccine candidate from the laboratory to the marketplace is a long, complex, arduous, and costly process (Dull and Bryan; IOM/NAS, 1985b; La Montagne and Curlin; Petricciani et al., 1989). The timetable for developing biologicals in the nineteenth century appeared to be very rapid, although it was not well documented (Dull and Bryan). After some preliminary tests in animals, vaccine candidates were readily injected into volunteers, with the timing based on the judgment of the scientist. Approval for clinical studies was not necessary, and studies were essentially conducted at the discretion of the investigator (personal communication, Robert Chanock, Chief, Laboratory of Infectious Diseases, NIAID, April 1993). There were no standardized requirements to be met. However, retrospective evaluation and critical debate among scientific peers was common (Dull and Bryan). Enhanced concern for human safety by the scientific community and the public and the increased complexity of scientific goals and techniques paved the way for the development of standards and regulations, which have effectively lengthened the process of vaccine development (ibid.). The length of time it takes from discovery to general clinical use of a vaccine remains quite variable (LaMontagne and Curlin; Petricciani et al., 1989). For example, the poliovirus was first identified in 1908, and a vaccine became available in 1955 (forty-seven years later), although, as others have pointed out, this was only six years after the poliovirus was successfully grown in cell culture; measles was identified in 1911 and a vaccine was licensed in 1963 (fifty-two years later); hepatitis B virus was first identified in the 1960s, was successfully transmitted to an animal model in 1973, and the first vaccine was licensed in 1981 (about seventeen years later) (LaMontagne and Curlin, p. 200). Vaccine candidates made by means of new molecular technologies are being developed rapidly. Before a license is granted for human use, however, both the process and the product are being scrutinized in greater detail than ever before.

> With the development of increasingly sophisticated analytical tools of molecular biology and immunology, vaccines derived from the newer technologies are receiving closer scrutiny at the regulatory and clinical levels than have vaccines derived from more classic strategies. . . . This trend . . . represents a formidable barrier for manufacturers to hurdle with respect to the licensing of safe and effective vaccines. (Ellis, 1988, p. 575)

Vaccine development is a long and multistep process which requires the integration of basic and clinical research. To begin with, basic research which can identify the causative agent and the components of the organism responsible for disease (infectivity, virulence, and pathogenicity) and characterize the host's response to infection is essential. The time-consuming and expensive research necessary to answer these questions is usually undertaken by academic or government researchers. Basic research is also necessary to develop or identify candidate vaccines, and to develop animal model systems for preclinical testing. Once the groundwork has been laid and a commercial manufacturer is interested, an efficient and reliable method must be found for producing the vaccine candidate in sufficient quantities for clinical testing and ultimately production. Historical examples of failure to conduct adequate preclinical testing of biologicals resulted in the endangerment of the lives of study participants and in public and scientific censure of the investigators (e.g., the polio vaccine trials in the 1930s of Kolmer, Brodie, and Parks) (Dull and Bryan).

Vaccines must be shown to be *safe, immunogenic,* and *protective* before being licensed. Ideally, an animal model which mimics the infection, clinical response, and immune response in humans is where evaluation of all three can occur before testing in humans begins. A first step in evaluation of a new vaccine is to test its ability to induce antibody in animals and then to test the effectiveness of these antibodies on the infectious agent in an *in vitro* laboratory assay (Petricciani et al., 1989). Unfortunately, for many vaccines this step has not been possible because of the lack of an appropriate animal model (e.g., measles) and/or the lack of an *in vitro* assay (e.g., hepatitis B). Because the human immune system is unique and some organisms infect humans in a specific way, it is difficult to find an animal model that simulates human infection and immune response; therefore testing of biologics is often a guessing game until the human model is used. Additionally, although nonhuman primates are often the animals that most closely resemble the human with respect to infection and response, they are very expensive, are in short supply, and require extensive long-term care, so their use is limited (see also chapter 4). Animal studies have been hindered not only by the inability to find appropriate models and limited availability but also by sociopolitical concerns about the use of animals in research.

Once a vaccine candidate induces neutralizing antibodies in animals, the animals can be challenged with the infecting agent to see if they are protected from infection or disease. Another important aspect of animal experimentation is the evaluation of potential toxicities from the vaccine candidate. If a candidate vaccine is shown to be safe in animals and able to protect a susceptible animal from infection, human testing can begin. The sponsor files an IND application with the FDA. To obtain the IND, appropriate regulatory requirements must be met, including purity of the product, qualifications of the investigators, safety and efficacy in animals or laboratory models, and approaches to clinical testing in human subjects.

Clinical research must demonstrate the safety and efficacy of the vaccine in humans. As guided by regulation, clinical research of vaccines is generally divided into phases which build on each other. Phase I studies evaluate general short-term safety and immunogenicity at various dose levels and sometimes for different routes of administration. These studies involve small numbers of subjects (now usually healthy adults) under close observation. Demonstration of safety is especially important when live attenuated vaccines are used. Despite close monitoring of participants, unexpected reactions will be observed only if they occur frequently. Phase II trials expand on the safety and immunogenicity evaluation, and also seek to determine the optimal immunization dose, route, and schedule. These trials involve larger numbers of subjects (usually hundreds) and attempt to include representatives of the population groups that will ultimately benefit from the use of the vaccine. Phase III clinical trials are controlled field trials which seek to establish the efficacy of the vaccine in preventing infection or disease. The final assessment of the value of potential vaccines for large-scale use can be made only by controlled field studies in humans (Kostrzewski), for only in humans can human safety, potency, and effectiveness be determined.

For scientific rigor, Phase III (and sometimes Phase II) clinical trials are controlled (i.e., some of the participants receive the investigational vaccine and some receive either another vaccine or a placebo), randomized (the designation of any given individual to the experimental group or the control group is by random assignment), and double-blind (neither the vaccinee nor the health care team knows whether the individual is receiving the experimental vaccine or the control). Random allocation of comparable individuals to the vaccine or the control groups is essential to ensure that there are no major biological, demographic, or behavioral differences between groups that could affect exposure to disease or the completeness of case ascertainment. All subjects should have the same risk of exposure to the disease. Field trials for efficacy involve large numbers of subjects identified as those in the target population at risk of infection and likely to benefit from utilization of an effective vaccine. The sample size is calculated based on the incidence rate of the infectious disease to which the vaccine is directed, the epidemiologic behavior of the organism, and the anticipated level of protection of the vaccine. Sample size for vaccine efficacy trials is at least in the hundreds, sometimes in the thousands or tens of thousands. The lower the incidence of the disease, the larger the sample needed to prove that the vaccine works, especially with a vaccine that has a relatively low protective efficacy. It is advisable that Phase III efficacy trials be conducted at more than one site and in more than one sample. If a vaccine is proven to be safe and efficacious, the sponsor applies to the FDA to have the product licensed. In addition to examining the data from the clinical evaluation of safety and efficacy in humans, the license application process includes review of all records of production and testing. The product itself is submitted for laboratory testing at the FDA, and CBER also provides on-site inspection of production facilities. If the FDA is satisfied that the product is pure, safe, and effective, a license is granted. The manufacturer of the vaccine must also be licensed.

Continued research and surveillance after licensure are also critical for confirming the safety and efficacy of vaccines. This stage is often referred to as Phase IV clinical research, or postmarketing surveillance. Continued observations and vigilance are required for a number of reasons. First of all, the effectiveness of a vaccine in general use may differ from that observed in controlled field trials, and/or undesirable side effects may not be manifested until hundreds of thousands or millions of persons have been vaccinated (IOM/NAS, 1985b; Kostrzewski). In addition, the duration of protection can sometimes be determined only by long-term follow-up and observation. After licensure, the manufacturer must submit data on each new production lot and send samples of vaccine to CBER for testing. CBER also periodically reinspects manufacturing facilities (IOM/NAS, 1985b, p. 22).

Recommendations for the use of vaccines in the U.S. are made by several advisory groups, especially the Advisory Committee on Immunization Practices (ACIP) of the U.S. Public Health Service (USPHS), the Committee on Infectious Diseases of the American Academy of Pediatrics, and the Committee on Immunizations of the American College of Physicians.

The value of a vaccine for the individual is based on a combination of its safety and efficacy. *Safety* is a relative term that basically means freedom from harmful side effects. By regulation, safety is defined as the "relative freedom from harmful effect to persons affected, directly or indirectly, by a product when prudently administered, taking into consideration the character of the product in relation to the condition of the recipient at the time" (U.S. 21CFR601.25(d)1). Immunogenicity means the ability of the vaccine to induce an immune response. Immunogenicity is usually evaluated by measuring the development of neutralizing and other functional antibodies against the organism as well as (more recently) by evaluation of the vaccine-induced cell-mediated responses. Since the goal of a vaccine is to induce a protective immune response in the individual, measuring immunogenicity is just the first step in the evaluation of efficacy. A vaccine must be able to induce a *protective* immune response, and this immune response must be appropriate to afford protection against the infection or disease.

Efficacy is the extent (usually expressed in percentages) of protection that the vaccine gives against the clinical manifestations of an infectious disease (Petricciani et al., 1989). It has also been defined as the "percent reduction in the incidence rate of the disease among vaccinated as compared to unvaccinated persons" (Begg and Miller, p. 181). A vaccine can be protective against infection itself or protective against the harmful effects of infection; i.e., it allows the establishment of subclinical infection but prevents clinical disease. Therefore, careful consideration of the case definition to be used in determining efficacy and how it is to be measured must be decided before efficacy trials begin.

Protective efficacy can be measured in different ways: the most usual and efficient method is a controlled clinical field trial which compares the rate of infection in a randomly assigned group of vaccinated persons to a control group who are unvaccinated or vaccinated with a control or placebo vaccine. Alternatively, although it is controversial, the efficacy of some vaccines has been tested initially by examining the immune response and clinical outcome of vaccinees challenged experimentally with either wild-type or vaccine virus (an unattenuated or attenuated version of the virus that is used to make the vaccine). Most, but not all, efficacy trials have been designed to evaluate individual protection against natural disease challenge (i.e., in the field). Other indications of efficacy include noting the reduction of the incidence of disease in a population after the introduction of vaccine into that population (but there can be other factors influencing incidence), and using a case control or cohort approach to compare the proportion of cases versus controls that are vaccinated (i.e., instead of prospectively comparing a vaccinated group with an unvaccinated control group, this method compares people with the disease with a control group and looks back to see how many of them have been vaccinated). This case-control method may be useful in long-term Phase IV surveillance of efficacy. Any vaccine's safety and efficacy can be influenced by the environment in which the vaccine is used. These influences may change depending on the persons, place, and time involved. Therefore, controlled clinical studies and field trials also attempt to evaluate differences in protective efficacy with respect to various host factors such as age, sex, immunocompetence, and the presence of other clinical diseases.

Clinical trials are absolutely required for the development and effective use of vaccines (LaMontagne and Curlin, p. 199). Without well-controlled and well-designed clinical trials, vaccine development would cease. History is full of examples of vaccines that were not accepted because of a lack of convincing evidence of their effect (e.g., A. Wright's typhoid fever vaccine), as well as of ineffective vaccines that were utilized at great expense for many decades because their effectiveness had never been rigorously tested (e.g., killed cholera vaccine).[10] The result has been unnecessary human suffering and cost, as well as diversion from potentially effective strategies of prevention or treatment. Enthusiasm about a new product and even compassion for people at risk can complicate and delay definitive evaluations of a vaccine's efficacy. Multiple causes, including sanitation, hygiene, behavior changes, environmental changes, and evolution or mutation of the infectious agent, can contribute to changes in the incidence of a given infectious disease. In some cases, just noting the decreased incidence of a disease could lead to unwarranted claims about the efficacy of a vaccine. Unsubstantiated belief in a vaccine's efficacy can also result in great difficulty in ever proving its real efficacy. An early fictional example of this phenomenon is Sinclair Lewis's Dr. Arrowsmith, who was never able to prove the efficacy of his bacteriophage because, in compassion, he gave it to everyone on a Caribbean island hit by an epidemic and left no controls for comparison.

The value of a vaccine to the community is based on (1) the needs (perceived and actual) of the community with respect to the control and prevention of a human disease; (2) sociopolitical attitudes which determine the acceptability, utilization, and relative value of the vaccine; (3) the cost of developing, testing, producing, and ultimately making the vaccine accessible to the target population; and (4) the safety and protective efficacy of the vaccine. New vaccines require an enormous investment of resources and extensive preclinical and clinical testing to prove their value. Because production of an effective vaccine depends on the ability to manufacture large quantities of a safe, immunogenic, and protective product, the interest of the private sector is essential. Industry must be willing to make an expensive investment for uncertain returns (Petricciani et al., 1989). Uncertainties include the size of the market (influenced by need and acceptability), who will pay for the vaccine, and liability risks. Vaccine development is also limited by finite funding for medical research and other research priorities, a litigious climate, a narrow public appreciation of the value of vaccines, and limited economic yield (profits) from vaccine sales, especially as compared to drugs (Peter, p. 982)

Vaccine development, testing, and use is a complex phenomenon whose history is replete with fascinating examples of success and failure. Several issues repeatedly surface in the literature:

1. Developing and using effective vaccines is extremely important in reducing the morbidity and mortality from infectious disease of large groups

of people. The impact of vaccination on the health of the world's peoples is difficult to exaggerate. No other modality, except sanitation and safe water, has had such a major effect on mortality reduction and population growth (Plotkin and Plotkin, 1988, p. 1).

2. Carefully conducted clinical trials are essential as a means of rigorously proving that a vaccine works and is safe. Without such proof, unnecessary harm and expense is incurred because of either lack of acceptance, which may hinder the use of an effective and useful vaccine, or unjustified acceptance, which may result in the wasteful use and risk of an ineffective vaccine, as well as impede finding a more effective one. Vaccine efficacy can be influenced by other factors, making a less rigorous research design problematic.

3. Even extremely effective and extremely safe vaccines have some margin of error. The risks and the failures can be influenced by a number of factors, some of which can be identified and minimized in the course of efficacy testing and/or postmarketing surveillance. The risks and the failures can also be exaggerated or misperceived, with negative consequences for vaccination in general. Perceptions of a vaccine's value and acceptability are influenced by the *incidence* of the infectious disease, the *perceived susceptibility* to and *severity* of the infectious disease, and the *perceived risk* and convenience of the vaccine itself.

4. Efficacy trials of vaccines are extremely difficult, costly, and complex to conduct:

•Historically, safety and preliminary efficacy of many vaccines was initially established in closed communities where infectious disease was often endemic, and where conditions, including exposure, were easy to control. Only after safety and some indication of efficacy was established in this way were large-scale efficacy trials in open communities attempted. (Some measure of the risks and benefits had already been obtained.) Current regulations limit human-subjects research with closed institutionalized populations because of their vulnerability. Establishing efficacy in the "field" is more difficult because of the interaction of other influences.

•The problem of what to use as a control is common. Many object to the use of placebo on the basis of the fact that proof of efficacy will be obtained only when the placebo group becomes infected or ill. It is also difficult to justify the use of a placebo control if the vaccine (for which efficacy is not clear) is already in wide use, or if there is already another effective vaccine in use. Yet, comparing a vaccinated group to historical controls may result in an inaccurate estimate of efficacy. Obtaining a sufficiently large sample with a sufficient incidence of disease in order to show a significant difference between the experimental and control group is a major challenge.

•The problem of how to measure efficacy is also common. If an antibody test or other immunologic response which indicates protection (for example, in a correlating *in vitro* test or animal model) can be identified and measured and not confounded by cross-reacting or preexisting antibodies, the measurement of efficacy may be relatively easy. Clinical evidence of infection or disease, although ultimately more meaningful, is more difficult to obtain in a reasonable time frame, requires reliable clinical resources, and is also confounded by a number of influences. Challenging volunteers under controlled conditions may be a more direct way to obtain an answer to efficacy, but challenging is acceptable only for certain (nonvirulent or treatable) pathogens, and even then is controversial.

5. Once a vaccine has been developed, shown to be safe and effective, and marketed, there are problems related to utilization. As Dr. Hilleman prophetically stated: "Vaccines will be considered useful only if they are used" (1985, p. 417). Differences in vaccine use are attributed to fear, apathy, cost, inconvenience, lack of information, a low priority on prevention, and inadequacies in health care delivery in general.

6. Politics, economics, scientific competition, media propaganda, and public attitudes have been and continue to be forces as powerful as scientific development and progress in influencing the development, testing, and utilization of vaccines.

CHAPTER TWO

▲
───
▼

Human-Subjects Research
and the Regulation of Drugs
and Biologicals

EARLY HISTORY

Research with human beings as subjects, also called clinical research, has a long history, as does the effort to define ethical codes and guidelines for its conduct. For many centuries the ethics of medicine or clinical research was sparingly discussed or written about. A few statements from various writers addressed research ethics, but these reflected the moral acuity of the commentators more than a shared sense of crisis or concern (Rothman, 1987b, p. 1196).

Legal concern with human experimentation can be traced back to the writings of an English court in 1767: "Many men skillful in their profession have frequently acted out of the common way for the sake of trying experiments . . . they have acted ignorantly and unskillfully" (Gray, 1975, p. 9). Doctors who experimented did so at their own risk.

William Beaumont, an American scientist, wrote in 1833 of the need for human experimentation when information is not otherwise available, but he also indicated the importance of methodologic soundness so that subjects are not exposed to risks for no scientific benefit. Beaumont pointed out the need for voluntary consent and the necessity to discontinue a project "when the subject becomes dissatisfied" (ibid., p. 9). Looking back today, one can see that Beaumont's ideas were quite ahead of his time.

Claude Bernard (1813–1878), a celebrated French physiologist and proponent of medical research, wrote in his *Introduction to the Study of Experimental Medicine*:

Physicians make therapeutic experiments daily on their subjects and surgeons perform vivesections daily on their subjects. Experiments, then, may be performed on men, but within what limits? It is our duty and right to perform an experiment on man whenever it can save his life, cure him, or gain him some personal benefit. The principle of medical and surgical morality, therefore, consists in never performing an experiment on man which might be harmful to him to any extent, even though the result may be highly advantageous to science, i.e., the health of others . . . and so among the experiments that may be tried on man, those that can only harm are forbidden, and those that may do good are obligatory. (Claude Bernard, as quoted in Altman, 1987, p. 102, and Veatch, 1987, p. 16)

The concepts of the value of clinical research in answering practical medical problems and the limits of research being protection of the individual are apparent. Interestingly, as Rothman points out, this quote has been repeated more frequently in the past twenty years than in the previous one hundred (1987b, p. 1194).

In 1916, Veressayev responded to experiments done on the nature and mode of transmission of gonorrhea and syphilis in which human volunteers were inoculated with discharges taken from other patients. He wrote, "It is high time . . . for society to take its own measures of self-protection against those zealots of science who have ceased to distinguish between their brothers and guinea pigs, without waiting for the faculty to emerge from its lethargy" (as quoted in Gray, 1975, p. 9). This statement appeared thirty years before Nuremberg, and almost sixty years before U.S. government regulations on clinical research.

Human experimentation began when the first doctor treated the first patients. However, until relatively recently, it was largely a trial-and-error process and not "scientific." For hundreds of years, physicians made little effort to formally coordinate knowledge, relying instead on intuition and personal experience. In the late seventeenth century, with the advent of medical journals, doctors began to systematically report cases (Altman, 1987, p. 14), first anecdotally, and later as more scientific case reports. For most of history, medical research was passive, including only observation and description of the natural course of events. The move to deliberate experimentation and intervention was more recent. Even so, experimental research for a long time was a "cottage" industry, conducted by a small number of physicians and scientists whose subjects usually included themselves and their families, and sometimes their neighbors and friends (Rothman, 1987b). The goal was usually to treat or prevent disease and thus to benefit the subject of the experiment. Examples include Edward Jenner's first test of a smallpox vaccine on his firstborn son and the neighbor's children and Louis Pasteur's first inoculation of Joseph Meister with his experimental rabies vaccine because young Joseph's death appeared otherwise inevitable.

In the 1890s, germ theory spurred research trials with hospital patients, but research still remained intimate and directly therapeutic, i.e., designed to benefit the subject him- or herself (Rothman, 1987b). During the nineteenth century, almost all medical practice was "experimental" in the sense that it was empirical and unproven. The most heroic, dangerous, and even lethal procedures were undertaken not as experiments but in an attempt to save lives (Howard-Jones, p. 456). Many of these unproven interventions were thought to be beneficial but instead were harmful or even lethal (for example, bloodletting as a treatment for cholera). A distinction between therapy and experimentation was hard to find, and research ethics was not a subject of much concern.

REGULATION OF DRUGS AND BIOLOGICALS

Until the early twentieth century there were no national regulations governing the sale of drugs in the U.S. Drugs, toxins, and potions were advertised directly to the public and purchased at will. Much of what was available was worthless, some toxic. Federal laws regulating the production and sale of drugs and biologics, and creating what we now know as the Food and Drug Administration (FDA), have all been written since the 1900s, most in response to catastrophe.

Although the need for care in the preparation and testing of vaccines was foreseen early in their development, it was not until major tragedies occurred that any action was taken to ensure public protection from unsafe products. In 1894 warnings about fraudulent and potentially unsafe preparations of diphtheria antitoxin were published in the *Journal of the American Medical Association*, and a few years later the director of the U.S. Hygienic Laboratory (predecessor of the National Institutes of Health) issued a statement warning about profiteers and diphtheria serum (Hopps, Meyer, and Parkman; IOM/NAS, 1985b). In the early 1900s, 13 children died as a result of receiving tetanus-contaminated diphtheria antitoxin (Hopps, Meyer, and Parkman, p. 577; IOM/NAS, 1985b, p. 16). The Biologics Control Act or Virus, Serum, Toxin Law was signed in July 1902, requiring evaluation and control of the purity and potency of any biological product (Hopps, Meyer, and Parkman).

Also in 1902, the Public Health and Marine Hospital Service was established. Its research arm, the Hygienic Lab, was expanded in 1930 and renamed the National Institutes of Health. Within the Hygienic Lab, the Biological Control Service assumed responsibility for regulation of smallpox vaccine and diphtheria and tetanus antitoxins (ibid.) and was authorized to inspect manufacturing establishments, issue and revoke licenses, and ensure the safety of the products. In 1937, this service was expanded and renamed the Laboratory of Biologics Control. U.S. Public Health Service Act 43, USC 262, 263, enacted in 1944, empowered the federal government to license biological products and their producers, inspect manufacturers, determine that the products were correctly labeled, and actually manufacture the biologics should the need arise (ibid.).

In 1906 the Pure Food and Drug Act was passed, forbidding manufacturers from making unsubstantiated claims on medicine labels (Arno and Feiden, p. 27). However, there was no mechanism for enforcing this rule, and no requirement for premarket approval, testing, or notification of "drugs." The Federal Bureau of Chemistry became the Food, Drug, and Insect Administration in 1927, and then in 1931 the Food and Drug Administration (Arno and Feiden). During the Depression in the United States, medical quackery was a common means of making a quick profit. Numerous scandals and tales of horror spurred repeated investigations and the introduction of legislation to impose more stringent controls. These proposed laws were continually struck down through the power of the pharmaceutical companies. In 1937, a substance called "Elixir Sulfonamide" caused the deaths of more than a hundred people because of the toxic solvent used. There had been no safety tests of the product before marketing. The ensuing public outcry led in 1938 to the passage of the Food, Drug, and Cosmetic Act, which made it illegal to market a drug until it was proven safe. This law coincided with the "golden age" of drug development, a period of explosive growth in pharmaceuticals, including penicillin and other antibiotics.

In 1955, in response to an incident in which 260 people who had received the Cutter polio vaccine developed paralytic polio and some died, the biologics control function of the U.S. Public Health Service (PHS) was expanded and the Division of Biologics Standards was established. In 1972 this division was transferred to the Food and Drug Administration and renamed the Bureau of Biologics; in 1982 it became the Office of Biologics Research and Review, and in 1987 the Center for Biologics Evaluation and Research (CBER). Authority for CBER exists in the PHS Act, Section 351, and in the Food, Drug, and Cosmetic Act. The mechanisms for implementing these statutes are in the Code of Federal Regulations, Title 21.

The "Utilitarian" Era of Human-Subjects Research

The turning point in human experimentation came during World War II. Many of the research practices established during the war shaped the future of clinical research. In the United States in 1941, President Roosevelt created an Office of Scientific Research and Development to oversee the work of two committees, one on weapons research and one on medical research. The goal of the Committee on Medical Research (CMR) was to plan and coordinate medical research primarily concerning the prevention and treatment of infectious diseases (Rothman, 1987b). During the war, clinical investigations became well-coordinated, extensive, and centrally funded. Experiments for the most part were designed to benefit not the subjects but others, for example, soldiers, who were at particular risk from certain infectious diseases. However, because research could not be conducted on the battlefield, institutions for the mentally impaired and prisons where infectious diseases were endemic were chosen as the primary sites for clinical research (Arno and Feiden; Rothman, 1987b). Experiments conducted under the auspices of the CMR included injecting mentally impaired inmates or prisoners with suspensions of bacteria or viruses in an attempt to find vaccines or treatments (Rothman, 1987b). In a University of Chicago study of malaria, approximately 500 prisoner "volunteers" were infected with malaria and then treated with an experimental drug, pentaquine (Altman, 1987; Rothman, 1987b). Although the study received little public attention, a *New York Times* article congratulated the prisoners for their contribution to the war effort. Another questionable experiment was the deliberate infection with malaria through blood transfusions of psychotic patients at a State Mental Hospital (Arno and Feiden, p. 25). There are many other examples of research which would never be approved, or even proposed, today. Participation in research had changed; no longer done primarily as a benefit to the subject, it was a burden and often risky, especially for disenfranchised populations (ibid., p. 24).

Nazi Germany brought the difficult issues in research with human beings to the attention of the public and medical/scientific communities. In the name of "experimentation," human torture and atrocities were performed on thousands of Jews and justified as being medical research. For example, Dr. Klaus Karl Schilling infected more than 1,000 prisoners at Dachau with malaria without their consent. More than 400 died from complications of the experimental antimalarial drugs, which were often given in excessive doses (Annas and Grodin). Despite the horror with which the world reacted to these atrocities, at the time of the Nuremberg trials there really was no formal code of ethics in medical research to which judges could hold the accused Nazi doctors accountable (Altman, 1987, p. 17). The "scientific experiments" exposed at the trials forced an examination of human research, its purposes, value, and limits. The medical profession was aware that serious breaches of ethics had also occurred in the past.

The Nuremberg Code was developed in 1949 as a ten-point code of human experimentation ethics, the concluding part of the judgment written after the trial of the Nazi doctors. It created the first widely recognized set of guidelines for the conduct of medical research in the world. This code recognized that human experimentation was valuable in that it could generate useful knowledge that was unobtainable by other means. It also categorically stated that the voluntary consent of the human subject is essential. Other points concerned the assessment and balancing of risk: "The degree of risk to be taken should never exceed that determined by the humanitarian importance of the problem to be solved"; all "unnecessary" physical and mental suffering and injury was to be avoided; and any anticipation of, or evidence of, injury, disability, or death to subjects meant the experiment should not be conducted or should immediately be terminated (taken from Annas and Grodin). Also stressed were the importance of preclinical data, adequate design, and scientifically qualified investigators.

Overall, the Nuremberg Code established that the ethical conduct of research must hold as its utmost priority the rights and welfare of the subject. Most subsequent codes and guidelines for the ethical conduct of human-subjects research have incorporated the basic ideas embodied in the Nuremberg Code.

In the wake of the Nuremberg trials, concern about voluntary informed consent was the central focus of biomedical research ethics. Subsequent codes adopted by individual countries and medical associations placed priority on the voluntary consent of the subject based on a full understanding of the risks involved. Disclosure of risk was seen as of primary importance in protecting the rights of the potential subject. Limitation of risk appeared to be secondary and was limited to cautioning the investigator that the risks of the research must be justified by the anticipated benefits, and that the risk of disabling injury or death was prohibited (President's Commission, p. 26).

Reliance on the investigator to determine that benefits and risks were reasonable was thought to be insufficient. During this period, "no routinely effective way existed to challenge the physicians' self-interest in research beyond informal consultations with colleagues" (Fletcher, 1983, p. 217). The informed consent of the individual participant did not adequately protect against investigator self-interest and partiality. A less explicit yet more fundamental and important question, whether the experiment should be done at all, was subject to an individual investigator's or involved group's discretion. It was noted that "the judgement of the investigator is not sufficient as a basis for reaching a conclusion concerning the ethical and moral set of questions" (NIH official, as quoted by ibid., p. 222). Consequently, policies requiring prior group review of proposed research began to be implemented as a means of enhancing impartiality.

GROWTH OF THE RESEARCH ENTERPRISE AND THE BEGINNING OF SOCIAL CONTROL

In the United States, the power, scope, and funding of biomedical research continued to expand enormously in the 1950s and 1960s. Support from the federal government and other sources for the conduct of research increased exponentially (Kieffer). The National Institutes of Health budget, for example, grew from less than half a million dollars before World War II, to $29 million in 1948, $1.25 billion by 1966 (Gray, 1975, p. 11), $4 billion in 1980 (President's Commission), and almost $9 billion in fiscal year 1992 (NIH Data Book, 1992). In addition, the value of medical research was increasingly recognized, and there were more medical students and physicians being educated to be investigators. Young scientists began to be judged by their investigative ability, as measured by publications (Kieffer). Also, there were new and compelling health problems amenable to investigation using human subjects (Beecher, p. 1354). During this period, the value of the randomized controlled clinical trial began to be recognized as the best means of providing a sound scientific basis for medical practice (National Research Council [NRC]).

When the Clinical Center of the NIH was opened in 1953, the need for principles and policies to protect subjects of research was recognized, and the first formal procedure for review of research proposals was developed (Fletcher, 1983, p. 222; Gray, 1975, p. 11). A document which called for group consideration of research projects was generated. It also included a discussion of what level of risk was acceptable and what information should be disclosed to subjects. These guidelines were revised but continued to pertain only to the intramural programs of research of the NIH (Gray, 1975, p. 11). In February 1966, the U.S. surgeon general issued regulations for human-subjects research in the "extramural" program, that is, all research supported by U.S. Public Health Service grants, contracts, and awards from the Department of Health, Education and Welfare (DHEW, now Department of Health and Human Services, DHHS). The requirements instituted by the USPHS in 1966 were based on the following general policy:

> PHS support of clinical research and investigation involving human beings should be provided only if the judgement of the investigator is subject to *prior review* by his institutional associates to assure an independent determination of the protection of the rights and welfare of the individual or individuals involved, of the appropriateness of the methods used to secure informed consent, and of the risks and potential medical benefits of the investigation. (Surgeon General, "Memo to Heads of Institutions Conducting Research with Public Health Service Grants," February 8, 1966, from Gray, 1975, p. 13)

This was the beginning of formalized requirements in the U.S. for prior review of research, with emphasis on the protection of the rights of the subject, informed consent, and the balancing of risks and benefits. In subsequent years, the requirement for prior independent review became codified, and the review "group" more diversified.

THE TUMULTUOUS 1960S

Two unrelated events during the early 1960s came together to transform the methods by which new medical technologies were researched and regulated. One involved the discovery in 1961–62 that thalidomide caused severe birth defects, and the other that researchers were still exposing their subjects to risk without necessarily obtaining their consent.

In the late 1950s, shocking stories of price gouging, stock manipulation, advertising fraud, and widespread deception on the part of the pharmaceutical industry, and multiple congressional hearings held on these violations at the request of Senator Kefauver, had failed to generate enough public interest to increase government control over the manufacture of drugs. Senator Kefauver had been pushing not only for control over the prices of drugs, but also for proof of effectiveness before marketing. The American Medical Association claimed that demanding proof of effectiveness before making a drug available for sale was a violation of a patient's freedom to choose (Arno and Feiden, p. 30). The tragedy that changed the tide was thalidomide. Thalidomide, widely used in Europe but unlicensed in the U.S., was thought to be an exceptionally safe sedative, ideal for pregnant women. The result was the births of thousands of children (most outside the U.S.) with severe and unusual deformities, most commonly phocomelia (hands attached to the shoulders and/or feet attached to the hips). These birth defects were unforeseeable because testing for teratogenicity was not considered necessary at the time (C. Levine, 1991a). The harm done was the result of inadequate research.

In 1962 the Kefauver-Harris amendments (also known as the Drug Amendments Act, P.L. 87–781, 21 U.S.C. 355) to the Food, Drug and Cosmetic Act of 1938 were passed in reaction to the tragedy (Katz, 1987; C. Levine, 1991a; Maloney; Veatch, 1987). This legislation required the U.S. Food and Drug Administration to impose new regulations on the clinical testing of experimental drugs and biologicals, mandating that they be shown through animal and human studies to be *efficacious* as well as *safe* before licensure. Previous regulations for drugs had called only for evidence of safety (Arno and Feiden; Hopps, Meyer, and Parkman; C. Levine, 1991a; NRC). Requirements included research on humans, not just on animals, and at the appropriate stage of development, because of differences in response by adults, children, and fetuses. Gaining the informed consent of the subject or his or her representative was mandatory, although requisite procedures for obtaining such consent were not specified. Procedural requirements for informed consent came in 1966 with the aforementioned USPHS policy.

The Kefauver-Harris amendments were a major impetus for the conduct of randomized clinical trials (RCTs), which soon became the accepted criterion for evaluating new drugs (NRC, p. 85). The legislation required "substantial evidence" of efficacy, including "adequate and well-controlled investigations, by experts qualified by scientific training and expertise." In accordance with the regulations subsequently established (codified in U.S. Code of Federal Regulations Title 21, part 312 or 21CFR.312), sponsors or investigators must submit an investigational new drug (IND) application to the FDA which includes evidence of completed *preclinical* testing for safety and efficacy as well as a justification and plan for human testing. The regulations divide human trials into three phases: Phase I to assess safety, Phase II to evaluate efficacy, and Phase III to compare the investigational drug to standard therapy or placebo, usually on a randomized, double-blind basis to determine effectiveness.

By regulation, vaccines are biologicals, not drugs, and the approval for licensing and marketing of vaccines comes under 21CFR.601, whereas new drug application regulations are found at 21CFR.314. However, regulations governing the *prelicensure testing* (i.e., clinical research) of biologicals are identical to those for drugs (21CFR.312). In the IND application requesting permission for clinical studies to be conducted with a given vaccine candidate, the sponsor must describe the composition, source, and manufacture of the product, and the methods used in testing it for safety (relative safety from harmful effects), purity (degree of freedom from extraneous matter), and potency (specific ability or capacity to effect a given result); provide a summary of all laboratory and animal testing; and provide a description of the proposed clinical study with the names and qualifications of each clinical investigator. The sponsor must then wait 30 days while the FDA reviews all the data to determine that human subjects will not be exposed to unwarranted risks. The product is assigned an IND number, and after approval from a local IRB and the documented informed consent of each participating subject, clinical studies may begin.

Clinical testing of vaccines usually consists of three separate phases. Phase I studies are the initial tests of the product in humans. Usually small numbers of normal subjects are included over a short period of time. The purpose is to test the properties of the biologic and the levels of toxicity. If toxicities are minimal and tolerable, Phase II studies are undertaken to obtain preliminary information on the effectiveness and relative safety of the vaccine. To this end, larger numbers of subjects, including some who will be eventual users of the vaccine, are included. Phase III studies involve more extensive testing to more fully assess safety and efficacy (Hopps, Meyer, and Parkman; La Montagne and Curlin; 21CFR.312).

In addition to the FDA regulations, important statements on the ethics of human experimentation were developed in the 1960s. Most notable was the Declaration of Helsinki (1964) by the World Medical Association. "A comprehensive international statement on the ethics of research involving human subjects" (Council for International Organizations of Medical Sciences [CIOMS], 1993, p. 9), the Declaration of Helsinki was written as a guide for the world's physicians involved in human-subjects research. It continued the Nuremberg emphasis on informed consent of the subject and a favorable balance of benefits to risks. Unless the importance of the objective was "in proportion" to the inherent risk to subjects, research was not justified. Unlike the Nuremberg Code, the Declaration of Helsinki distinguished between clinical research combined with patient care (therapeutic or clinical research) and nontherapeutic research involving human subjects (which was called "nonclinical" biomedical research). This was the first formal distinction between experimentation which might also be beneficial to the subject and experimentation purely for the generation of clinically useful knowledge with no expected benefit for the individual subject. The Declaration is called the "fundamental document in the field of ethics in biomedical research and has had considerable influence on the formulation of international, regional, and national legislation and codes of ethics" (CIOMS, 1993, p. 9). It has since been revised several times (Tokyo, 1975; Italy, 1983; and Hong Kong, 1989).

The other major event of the 1960s, widespread concern about the abuse of human subjects of medical research, was generated primarily by the exposition of several studies which breached accepted ethical standards of clinical research and were seen as flagrant abuses of human beings in the name of science.

In 1966, a landmark article written by the prestigious Dr. Henry Beecher and published in the *New England Journal of Medicine* clearly aroused the concern of the medical profession and subsequently public interest in protecting people from the abuses of research. Beecher wrote about 22 research experiments which violated the rights and dignity of the involved subjects and put people at considerable risk. Beecher argued that the "gain anticipated from an experiment must be commensurate with the risk involved. An experiment is ethical or not at its inception" (1966, p. 1360). He concluded that two factors are essential for the ethical conduct of research: the informed consent of the subject, and an "intelligent, informed, conscientious, compassionate, responsible investigator" (ibid.). Others had already recognized the necessity of prior independent review rather than reliance on the judgment and integrity of the investigator.

Two books, *Human Guinea Pigs* (Pappworth, 1967) and *Experimentation with Human Beings* (Katz, 1972), also drew attention to abuses. In many of the cases cited, subjects were exposed to a variety of risky procedures not intended to benefit them. Subjects included newborns, infants and children (healthy and diseased), pregnant women, prisoners, patients undergoing surgery, the mentally impaired, the aged, the critically ill, and the dying.

Several experiments received considerable attention in the lay and scientific press. At the Jewish Chronic Disease Hospital in Brooklyn, two physician investigators injected cultured cancer cells into debilitated elderly patients under their care without informing the patients of the contents of the injection or obtaining their consent. Three young staff physicians resigned rather than participate in this experiment (Fletcher, 1983). The investigators were found to be "guilty of fraud or deceit . . . and of unprofessional conduct" and put on probation for one year (President's Commission, p. 31). At the Willowbrook State School, investigators injected hepatitis B virus into mentally retarded children, with the consent of their parents, in order to study the natural history of the disease and to explore avenues for preventive vaccines. The investigators were harshly criticized for subjecting children to unknown and unjustified risks without benefit (Krugman, 1986; Krugman, Giles, and Hammond, 1971; Krugman and Giles; President's Commission; and others).

The Tuskegee syphilis study, conducted by the USPHS, recruited poor black males who had naturally acquired syphilis to voluntarily participate in a study of the natural course of infection and disease in exchange for free medical care and free burials. Some of the men were followed for more than forty years (Caplan, 1992b; President's Commission). During the course of the study, penicillin was found to be an effective therapy in early syphilis, yet it was never offered to the Tuskegee subjects (A. Brandt, 1978b; Edgar; King;

Jones; Thomas and Quinn). Pressured by exposure in the national press in the early 1970s, the U.S. DHEW established an ad hoc committee to examine the study. The panel concluded that the Tuskegee study was "ethically unjustified at its inception" (President's Commission, p. 37), finding that the program had not provided for informed consent, lacked a written protocol, and was questionably designed (Fletcher, 1977, p. 102; Katz, 1987). Many have also concluded that the Tuskegee study was racist by design (A. Brandt, 1978b; Edgar; King; Jones; Thomas and Quinn). The ad hoc panel also reviewed U.S. DHEW policies and guidelines and expressed concern about overrepresentation of biomedical professionals in the regulatory process, vagueness of the guidelines, loopholes in the consent procedures, insufficient attention to vulnerable subject populations, and neglect of the need for continuing review and the absence of effective enforcement procedures (President's Commission, p. 38). The panel members recommended the creation of a national board to reexamine human experimentation (Caplan, 1992).

Despite the Nazi experience, the Nuremberg Code, the Declaration of Helsinki, and other attention to the problem, experiments which clearly breached the ethics of human research were still being performed. This concern with the abuse of human subjects coincided in the U.S. with the civil rights movement of the 1960s, with its strong emphasis on the rights of individuals. The late 1960s and early 1970s, the era of the Vietnam War and Watergate, were a time of general mistrust and disillusionment with public agencies and government officials—a time when concern about privacy and freedom of the individual from unwarranted government control was significant.

THE WORK OF THE
NATIONAL COMMISSION

The expositions and public attention led to an intense debate about the ethics of human experimentation, and to a series of hearings held by the Subcommittee on Health of the U.S. Senate Committee on Labor and Public Welfare. Based in large part on these hearings, the U.S. Congress in 1974 passed the National Research Act (P.L. 93–348), which required the independent review of all research by an institutional review board (IRB) before it was funded, and also established the National Commission for the Protection of Human Subjects of Biomedical and Behavioral Research (Maloney; NRC; Veatch, 1987). The act established the commission as advisory to the U.S. DHEW and stipulated that it was to be replaced by a long-term National Advisory Council. Between 1975 and 1978, the National Commission published seventeen reports and numerous appendix volumes (Caplan, 1992b). Included were special reports on the use of human fetuses, prisoners, children, and the institutionalized mentally infirm; a report on institutional review boards recommending their continued use; and a report on basic ethical principles guiding human-subjects research (referred to as the Belmont Report) (Veatch, 1987, p. 95). To date, probably the single most influential body in the United States involved with the protection of human research subjects was the National Commission. Although it was formally dissolved in October 1978, its activities were taken over for a few years by other federal commissions and agencies. The President's Commission for the Study of Ethical Problems in Medicine and Biomedical and Behavioral Research actively assumed such a role in 1980. The Ethics Advisory Board of the U.S. DHEW (1978–80) initially played a role in continuing the work of the National Commission, focusing to a large extent on *in vitro* fertilization. The National Commission not only produced a thorough examination of the issues, but also served as "an important model for future efforts in ethics and public policy" (Veatch, 1987, p. 96).

The National Commission's *Belmont Report: Ethical Principles and Guidelines for the Protection of Human Subjects of Research* (1979) was an attempt to summarize the ethical principles basic to the conduct of research with human subjects. The commission and others felt that the Nuremberg and other existing codes were often "inadequate to cover complex situations at times when they come into conflict, and . . . frequently difficult to interpret or apply" (National Commission for the Protection of Human Subjects of Biomedical and Behavioral Research, p. 3). In writing the Belmont Report, the commission identified broader ethical principles to provide "a basis on which specific rules could be formulated, criticized, and interpreted" (ibid.). The report described three underlying principles for the evaluation of human-subjects research: respect for persons, beneficence, and justice. The three principles are described conceptually, and their application to the processes of informed consent, risk/benefit assessment, and selection of subjects is discussed. The report emphasized the distinction between "research," an activity designed to develop or contribute to generalizable knowledge, and "practice," an activity designed to provide diagnosis, prevention, or therapy to an individual for the purpose of enhancing the well-being (benefit) of that individual.

Respect for persons was described as including both treating individuals as autonomous agents and protecting those incapable of self-determination. The commission recognized, however, that in many situations, competing claims derived from this single principle can come into conflict. For example, should prisoners be given the "opportunity to volunteer" for research or "protected" from undue influence, subtle or otherwise? The principle of respect for persons requires that subjects who participate in research do so voluntarily and with adequate information, i.e., give their voluntary informed consent. The consent process has three elements: information, comprehension, and voluntariness. The commission recommended the use of a standard of the "reasonable volunteer" to determine the extent and nature of information to be given, such that "persons, knowing that the procedure is neither necessary for their care nor perhaps fully understood, can decide whether they want to participate in the furthering of knowledge" (National Commission, 1979, p. 6). Investigators are responsible for determining that subjects have comprehended the information, and therefore they are obligated to provide information to subjects or their surrogates in a way that facilitates comprehension. Recognizing that influencing factors are hard to eliminate or even sometimes to identify, the commission affirmed that consent is valid only if given voluntarily.

Beneficence is defined in the Belmont Report as an obligation both to do no harm and to maximize possible benefits and minimize possible harms. It is recognized that in research, risks must sometimes be accepted in order to *learn* what is harmful and what is beneficial. The trick is to determine when it is justifiable to seek certain benefits despite the risks, and when the benefits should be foregone because of the anticipated risks. The investigator is obligated by beneficence to maximize benefits and minimize risks for a given research project, while society is obligated to maximize long-term benefits and minimize long-term risks from the improvement of knowledge and the development of novel health care procedures through research. The commission applies the principle of beneficence to the assessment of risks and benefits to determine if the research in question is justified, properly designed, and accurately presented to prospective subjects. This assessment is concerned with the probabilities and magnitudes of possible harms and anticipated benefits to the individual and to others (family, society). Many kinds of possible harms and benefits (physical, psychological, social, legal, economic) should be considered. In general, potential risks to subjects should be outweighed by benefits to subjects and to society. If no benefit to the individual is anticipated, then benefit to others must be a strong factor, risk to the subject must be minimal, and the individual's rights must be protected. Assessment of risks and benefits can be made only through a thorough and systematic examination of information about all aspects of the research and alternatives. The commission also mentions the risk (or "loss of substantial benefits") of not doing research.

Justice, as described by the commission, is the principle of distributive justice, i.e., fairness in the distribution of the benefits and burdens of research. They cite several historical examples in which vulnerable populations were burdened with the risk of being subjects of research, the results of which predominantly benefited others. The principle of justice is described as particularly relevant to the *selection* of research subjects. Subjects should not be selected disproportionately from groups who will not benefit from the subsequent application of the research. The just selection of subjects pertains to individuals—potentially beneficial research should not be offered only to favored patients and risky research to "undesirable" patients—and to society—groups of subjects should be selected fairly, not based on societal biases, easy availability, or vulnerability (National Commission, 1979). Additionally, justice demands that the fruits of research supported by public funds be distributed fairly, "not only to those who can afford them" (ibid., p. 5).

The emphasis of the work of the National Commission was on the need to *protect* individuals from the potential dangers of research. Volunteering to participate in research was viewed as a burden or sacrifice performed for the public good (NRC, p. 88). The commission affirmed the importance of scientific research and clinical investigation as good for society, but identified ethical principles by which research should be evaluated and mechanisms applied to protect subjects from possible harm. The potential benefits to society from research were limited by the need to protect the rights and welfare of the individual research subject. The goal of research was *not* benefit to the individual. Although possible benefit to the individual was a necessary part of the equation in order to justify research, and individuals often did benefit from participation, regulations were based on the assumption that being a research subject was a burden. Individuals needed protection from too much burden, and the burden should be distributed as equitably as possible.

The National Commission wielded considerable power in guiding the formulation of regulations. The U.S. DHEW (now DHHS) was required by statute to act upon commission recommendations by reworking them into regulations. The department developed proposed and final regulations, and published them in the Federal Register. These regulations, "Protection of Human Subjects," were codified in the U.S. Code of Federal Regulations in 1981 (US 45CFR.46). Since then there have been a few modifications and revisions, most recently in June of 1991.

Federal regulations require that all research involving human subjects and conducted or funded by the DHHS be reviewed and approved by an IRB composed of at least five members of varying backgrounds (45CFR.46.107). There must be at least one member with scientific concerns and one with nonscientific concerns, members must be of both sexes, and one member must be unaffiliated with the institution. The IRB can approve the proposed research by a majority vote, require modifications, or disapprove the research. Approval should be based on the following criteria:

1. Risks to subjects are minimized by using procedures that are consistent with sound research design. In other words, what the investigator proposes to do has a good possibility of answering the question with minimal risk to the subject (beneficence).

2. The "risks are reasonable in relationship to anticipated benefits, if any, to the subject and the importance of the knowledge that may reasonably be expected to result" (45CFR.46.111 (a)(2)) (beneficence).

3. Subject selection is equitable (justice).

4. Informed consent will be sought from each subject or legally authorized representative and will be documented (respect for persons).

5. Data will be monitored to ensure safety (beneficence).

6. The privacy and confidentiality of the subjects will be protected (respect for persons).

7. Additional safeguards are included when subjects are vulnerable to coercion or undue influence ("such as children, prisoners, pregnant women, mentally disabled persons, and economically or educationally disadvantaged") (45CFR46.111) (respect for persons, and justice).

Other subparts of part 46 of CFR Title 45 specify additional protection for research involving fetuses and pregnant women (Subpart B), prisoners (Subpart C), and children (Subpart D) as subjects.

In 1975, the secretary of DHEW established a task force to study compensation of persons injured during participation in research. It recommended that human subjects who suffer physical, psychological, or social injury in the course of research conducted or supported by PHS should be recompensed. The practical problem of developing a compensation scheme was later assigned to the President's Commission, which issued a report in 1982. To date, no mechanism exists to compensate subjects injured as a result of participation in research. Subsequent to the President's Commission report, it was determined that nonnegligible injury resulting from participation in research was so infrequent that the development of a program was not warranted.

The President's Commission, established in 1978 by P.L. 95–622, began in 1980 to take over some of the work of the National Commission. The President's Commission had two main purposes: to finish and expand upon topics addressed by the National Commission, and to address additional topics such as allocation of health care, and review and monitor implementation of existing regulations on research in all federal agencies (Maloney). The President's Commission compiled nine reports before its end in March 1983. Those that pertained to human-subjects research included *Implementing Human Research Regulations: The Adequacy and Uniformity of Federal Rules and Their Implementation*, which recommended that all federal agencies adopt DHHS regulations 45CFR part 46 governing the conduct of human-subjects research, and urged the secretary of DHHS to establish an office to coordinate and monitor the implementation of these regulations. A Proposed Model Federal Policy for the Protection of Human Subjects of Research was developed by an ad hoc committee, modified by the Office of Science and Technology Policy (OSTP), and codified in the regulations in June 1991 (Dickens, Gostin, and Levine; Federal Register, June 18, 1991). This Common Rule also addresses the approval of foreign research that may follow different procedures to protect human subjects. Review must find these procedures in compliance with the Declaration of Helsinki or another internationally accepted code of ethics (Dickens, Gostin, and Levine). Two other relevant reports were *Compensating for Research Injuries: The Ethical and Legal Implications of Programs to Redress Injured Subjects* and *Whistleblowing in Biomedical Research: Policy and Procedures for Response to Reports of Misconduct* (Helm).

THE STATUS OF HUMAN-SUBJECTS RESEARCH AND DRUG REGULATION ON THE EVE OF THE HIV EPIDEMIC

Between the 1940s and the 1980s, clinical research had seen a remarkable expansion in public support and funding; a large increase in highly educated investigators who functioned under considerable pressure to investigate and publish; the availability of increasingly more sophisticated technologies to use in research with the associated uncertainties regarding long-term risks and benefits; and an increasingly attentive and scrutinizing public with quicker access to information about science and clinical trials. Concurrently, a number of widely circulated and accepted codes of ethics concerning research had been developed. In the U.S., regulations were in place which required IRB review, informed consent, the balancing of risks and benefits, and scientific rigor in demonstrating the safety and efficacy of new products for diagnostic, therapeutic, or prophylactic use. An increasingly voluminous body of literature on the ethics of clinical research generally accepted the three underlying principles identified in the Belmont Report as "non-controversial" and relevant to clinical research (Ackerman, 1992; Arno and Feiden; Beauchamp and Childress; Brett and Grodin; Carter, McCarthy, and Wichman; Freedman, 1987b; C. Levine, 1988; R. Levine, 1986; Macklin and Friedland; Shorr; Walters; and others). Criticism of the Belmont Report was limited to commentary on the difficulty of applying the principles, the lack of guidance as to how to reconcile conflicts between principles, and the lack of a unifying theory upon which the principles were based (see Beauchamp and Childress; De Grazia; Marshall; and others). A major shift had occurred from an ethics of research in the U.S. which was "frankly and unashamedly utilitarian" (Rothman, 1987b, p. 1198) during World War II, to an ethics of research which recognized primarily the inviolability of the individual research subject and sought to protect his/her rights and welfare. It was generally agreed that for research to be ethically acceptable, reviewers and regulators must judge that several rules are satisfied: subjects must give voluntary informed consent; the study design and prior animal experimentation should minimize risk and offer a high probability of generating useful knowledge; the probable benefits to subjects and/or society must outweigh risks to the subject; the selection of subjects must be just; and the investigators must be qualified (Beauchamp and Childress, p. 64; Gray, p. 7). Although there seemed to be some consensus about the major issues, controversy about the drug development process continued, and the ethics of "human subjects research was not a closed topic" (C. Levine, 1991a).

When the HIV/AIDS epidemic appeared in the early 1980s, a transition had already begun from an emphasis on protecting subjects to an emphasis on the need for more rapid approval of potentially helpful products (C. Levine, 1988 and 1991a; Shorr). The HIV epidemic accelerated this transition and produced a sustained attack on the premises and structure of drug regulation and human experimentation. Some of the claims in fact challenged the ethical justification for the regulation of drug approval and clinical research (Shorr).

In addition to the impact of the AIDS epidemic, other forces in the 1980s were creating a resurgence of interest in research ethics, including the dramatic increase in international collaborative research, and a realization by some that existing guidelines had focused on the burdens and protection of the individual involved in research, ignoring the communities involved (Dickens, Gostin, and Levine; Gostin, 1991). Community rights and welfare and protecting communities from the burdens of research, issues particularly relevant to large-scale studies of vaccines, had received almost no attention.

The Council for International Organizations of Medical Sciences (CIOMS) in conjunction with the World Health Organization in 1982 issued "Proposed International Guidelines for the Conduct of Biomedical Research." Previous codes, such as the Nuremberg Code and the Declaration of Helsinki, had focused on the primacy of the individual, providing little guidance for applying principles in non-Western settings where cultural and moral values are less individualistic. The CIOMS/WHO-proposed guidelines were concerned with application of the principles to the "special circumstances of many technologically developing countries" (Christakis and Panner, p. 1215). These guidelines were more comprehensive than Helsinki, were recommended worldwide, and have achieved broad acceptance in many countries throughout the world (Dickens, Gostin, and Levine, p. 158). Nonetheless, disagreement still exists regarding whether ethical principles and guidelines governing clinical research can and should be universally applicable or locally specific (Christakis and Panner). The CIOMS, recognizing that neither the Declaration of Helsinki nor their own 1982 guidelines adequately addressed population-based research, including large-scale intervention trials of vaccines or drugs, issued *International Guidelines for Ethical Review of Epidemiological Studies* in 1991. In 1993 the CIOMS also published *International Ethical Guidelines for Biomedical Research Involving Human Subjects* (a revision of their 1982 guidelines) to reflect changes in the perception and practice of clinical research.

THE IMPACT OF THE HIV EPIDEMIC

Primarily because of the HIV epidemic, the 1980s saw dramatic changes in both attention and attitudes toward and the conduct and regulation of clinical research and drug development in the United States (Broder; Cooper; Edgar and Rothman; Freedman, 1992; Kessler; C. Levine, 1988 and 1991a; NRC; Rothman and Edgar, 1992; Shorr; and others).

> The AIDS epidemic would severely strain virtually every assumption of what had become (over 20 years) the guiding, orthodox assumptions regarding clinical research and the regulation of new drugs. Every aspect of the process by which pharmacologic agents were identified, evaluated, regulated, and allocated would be tested by the exigencies of epidemic disease. Questions basic to the epistemologic foundations of biomedicine . . . would all be subject to debate and reevaluation. In this respect, the epidemic (HIV) has already had a profound social impact on science and medicine. (NRC, pp. 89–90)

THE CRITICISMS

The HIV epidemic brought out much criticism of the procedures for conducting clinical trials and regulating the approval of new drugs and therapies. The entire process by which drugs move from the laboratory to the marketplace came under unprecedented public scrutiny. Academic institutions and government agencies involved in drug development and approval became the targets of political protests and accusations.

The FDA was accused by AIDS activists of being too slow, restrictive, and paternalistic. The FDA had had many critics before AIDS, predominantly among the pharmaceutical industry and academicians, who claimed that the required extensive and expensive use of the controlled clinical trial slowed the development of potentially beneficial drugs ("drug lag") and decreased incentives for companies to develop new drugs (Rothman and Edgar, 1992). As a regulatory agency, the FDA was committed to scientific rigor and consumer protection. That commitment plus a chronic shortage of resources made the FDA process slow and cumbersome, more adept at keeping bad drugs off the market than at making good ones accessible (Arno and Feiden). These criticisms were not of the FDA's role in protecting the consumer, nor of the importance of proving safety and efficacy through controlled trials, but of the overly long and expensive process of obtaining drug approval. It took a few years and a few million dollars to adequately prove a drug's value before the 1962 Kefauver amendments, but in the 1970s about ten years and $100 million was the norm (Edgar and Rothman, p. 119). Consequently, potentially beneficial drugs were not available for long periods of time, and companies had decreased incentives to find new drugs, especially for diseases that were sufficiently rare that it would not pay to produce a treatment for them. The FDA also had a reputation for being critical, suspicious, and nondirective with pharmaceutical companies, rather than collaborative. People with HIV and their advocates reacted with fury to the slow pace of drug development. They argued that the FDA should be proactive, not reactive; that the government's role should be to maximize choice, not to usurp people's right to make decisions. They rejected the paternalism and risk-averse attitudes of the FDA, claiming that as long as a drug is safe, it should be available to anyone who wants it, even if it is medically worthless. In criticizing and calling for changes at the FDA, there was a "curious overlapping of the interests of sick gay men with the pharmaceutical industry which had long complained of the FDA's proclivity for caution" (Arno and Feiden, p. 34), as well as an "unusual political alliance between the antiregulation Reagan and Bush administrations and gay rights activists" (Annas, 1990, p. 184). However, at least in part, the industry's motives were profit and the administration's motives were libertarian anti-regulationism, while patients were motivated by desperation and fear. Academicians, policymakers, patient advocates, and ethicists sought a middle ground, a better balance between the duty to ensure safe and effective drugs (protection of the public) and the duty to make potentially beneficial agents available on a timely basis.

Many in the HIV community also rejected the traditional methods of conducting clinical trials. They claimed that trials were too restrictive and slow, that the exclusion of certain groups from participation was discriminatory, and that the methodology, especially the use of placebo controls, was unfair, unnecessary, and even criminal (Arno and Feiden; Rothman and Edgar, 1992; C. Levine, 1991a; NRC; and others).

The HIV epidemic created a vocal constituency of individuals who were eager to take risks with unproven therapies. Patients wanted to make their own decisions, arguing that risk could be defined only in a very specific personal and social context (NRC). The search for an effective treatment became an obsession for some HIV-infected persons, who volunteered for every study and tried every substance rumored on the street to be helpful. Fads and quackery were and are common, with many unfounded claims for various sham or untried therapies. People joked about the "drug-of-the-month-club," as the community's hopes surged with one promising substance after another. The AIDS underground, feeling that the medical establishment was unable or unwilling to give them the drugs they wanted, took matters into their own hands. Drug smuggling and bootlegging became commonplace. Project Inform, a San Francisco–based AIDS advocacy group, published a detailed guide on importing two experimental antiviral drugs (ribaviran and isoprinosine) from Mexico (Arno and Feiden, p. 65). Buyers' clubs were created where otherwise unavailable drugs could be purchased. Recipes for concocting homemade versions of certain "beneficial" substances (such as AL721) were published in gay publications across the nation (Arno and Feiden). As one activist said, "The underground has become mainstream and this is inexcusable" (Derek Hodel, as quoted by ibid., p. 68). In perhaps the most dramatic example of taking action, Project Inform planned and carried out its own clinical trial of Compound Q without applying for an IND from the FDA or obtaining the review of an IRB. These trials were highly criticized. Several people died, presumably as a result of Compound Q, and Project Inform later did submit an IND application to the FDA.

AIDS activism may be best understood in its historical context. In many ways it followed from the strong gay rights movement of the 1970s, in which an increasingly visible gay community fought discrimination, insisted on a presence in public discourse and consciousness, and struggled to control their own institutions.[11] A gradual change in the balance of the health care provider/patient relationship from paternalism to respect for the autonomy of the patient, the legal codification of informed consent, the patients' rights movements, and growing skepticism by patients about medical and scientific authority all set the stage for the demands of the AIDS activists. Activists, especially gay community groups, were involved in political and community organizing from the beginning of the AIDS epidemic in 1981. Their early efforts were primarily directed toward minimizing discrimination against gays and against people with AIDS, and in expanding access to health care. Attention was also given to the needs and rights of patients to refuse life-sustaining therapy and to receive compassionate, low-cost care in a variety of settings. Their focus on, and criticism of, drug development surfaced with Rock Hudson's journey to Paris in 1985 to receive the experimental antiviral drug HPA-23. (Interestingly, HPA-23 was shortly thereafter shown to be ineffective, and another investigational antiretroviral drug, suramin, was shown to actually be harmful, supporting the importance of carefully controlled clinical trials.)

By early 1986, the safety and promise of another experimental antiviral drug, zidovudine (AZT), had been demonstrated in Phase I trials, and a multicenter placebo-controlled Phase II trial was initiated. When a difference in survival between the AZT group and the control group was noted by the Data and Safety Monitoring Board, the trial was stopped prematurely and AZT was given to all participants. The FDA hurried it through the approval process, and it was licensed in early 1987 (only about a year from the beginning of clinical research with the drug). In the words of Dr. Samuel Broder, who was responsible for the preclinical and early clinical research on AZT for HIV infection, "For drug development, that is the speed of light" (as quoted in Arno and Feiden, p. 46).

Around the same time, AIDS activists visibly fought for patient empowerment and refused to be "passive victims." These groups showed their willingness and adeptness at fighting the system and taking matters into their own hands. The AIDS Coalition to Unleash Power (ACT-UP) was started in New York in 1987 and eventually grew into an "angry, loud, and highly effective political pressure group" (ibid., p. 61) in numerous cities around the country. ACT-UP and other activist groups became increasingly visible and began to focus their efforts on the development and approval of drugs.

In addition to complaints about the exigencies and pace of the drug approval process, activists were highly critical of the accepted methods of conducting clinical trials. They argued that strict eligibility criteria, scientifically defended by the need to minimize confounding variables, led to a sample which was unrepresentative of those who ultimately needed the drug (such as the very sick, those with multiple opportunistic infections, and substance abusers) and was harmful to participants because criteria sometimes precluded the use of other drugs. The exclusion from clinical trials of groups because of "vulnerability," such as children or women of childbearing age, or because of perceived lack of cooperation, for example, active substance abusers, was called discriminatory. Rather than protecting groups from exploitation as research subjects, underinclusion or limited access was seen as exploitative, harmful, and unjust. Participation in clinical trials was seen as a benefit, so those denied access were being harmed. Some perceived participation not only as a benefit but as a right. Patients begged, bribed, lied, and cheated in order to participate in clinical trials (Arno and Feiden). ACT-UP claimed that "A Drug Trial Is Health Care Too" (Annas, 1990). The distinction between the goals of research and of health care was denied.

Interestingly, as gay activists were claiming a right to access to clinical trials, other groups, particularly minorities, continued to resist participation. African American spokespersons explained that this was based on an inherent distrust of authorities, government, and the research system, in large part due to the legacy of Tuskegee. For a surprisingly large number of African Americans, the HIV epidemic is perceived as a deliberate genocidal conspiracy against the African American community. Clinical trials of toxic drugs are viewed as just a part of that conspiracy (A. M. Brandt, 1988; Des Jarlais and Stephenson; King; Jones; Thomas and Quinn).

The tradition of conducting clinical trials at tertiary care facilities and in academic institutions (usually done because of the availability of expertise, skilled personnel, IRBs, laboratory facilities, and other supports) was also challenged. AIDS advocates argued that studies could be carried out more efficiently, more equitably, and with increased compliance if community physicians and community health care sites were involved, and if members of the affected community were involved in the processes of planning, designing, and evaluating the research. Scientists countered that the value of the conclusion of any study is only as good as the study design and the quality of the data collected; therefore, giving up the expertise and the careful conditions of the experienced tertiary care facilities potentially compromised the science (Richman).

Activists also challenged the orthodoxy of control groups in randomized clinical trials, especially placebo-controlled trials. Protesters held placards with statements such as "I died on placebo." They claimed that many people, but especially those with life-threatening illnesses, would willingly risk the unknowns of a potentially beneficial investigational drug. (This argument had been used before by cancer patients and cancer researchers; see Rothman and Edgar, 1991.) Subjects involved in placebo-controlled trials were encouraged by the community to have their "drug" analyzed, and if they were on placebo to withdraw from the study and find an active drug. Active drugs from clinical trials, as well as other substances perceived to be beneficial, were relatively easy to find (although often expensive) through buyers' clubs. Activists called for relinquishing the dependence on randomized clinical trials and utilizing other designs for clinical research.

In addition, AIDS activists demanded access to information about clinical trials and preliminary data as soon as it was available. Scientists argued that preliminary data are often misleading, and completing the trial as planned increases the validity and usefulness of the data. Activists accused scientists of hiding information until it could be used for their own self-aggrandizement. The gay community especially had produced an extremely well-informed pool of potential and actual research subjects. They demanded information based on the right of the research subject to be informed in order to make choices about continuing or discontinuing participation in research. Many AIDS advocacy groups circulate their own newsletters or other documents reporting details of clinical trials and preliminary preclinical and clinical data from multiple sources. Examples include *AIDS Treatment News* and the American Foundation for AIDS Research (AmFAR) *AIDS/HIV Experimental Treatment Directory*.

THE ETHICS OF RANDOMIZED CLINICAL TRIALS (RCTS)

Although the randomized clinical trial was widely accepted as the gold standard of clinical research, it had not been as universally utilized (see, among others, Chalmers, 1981; Rothman and Edgar, 1991; NRC). Even the FDA does not insist on placebo-controlled studies. In the regulations which require evidence of "adequate and well-controlled studies" (21CFR.314.126), five types of controls are recognized as acceptable, including historical controls under "special circumstances" (21CFR.314.126). A body of literature exists, much of which predates AIDS, which debates the ethical pros and cons of randomized controlled clinical trials.[12] The major ethical controversies include the following questions:

1. What is the justification for doing a randomized clinical trial? It is generally agreed that an investigator must have a true null hypothesis or "clinical equipoise" (Freedman, 1987b) in order to justify beginning an RCT. There must not exist conclusive evidence to demonstrate that the experimental drug is better than (and/or less harmful than) the active or placebo control; otherwise the control group would be assigned to no or less benefit (or more harm). Some argue that equipoise is impossible to maintain as soon as there are even preliminary data on efficacy.

2. Does randomization violate the subject's autonomy, and is the appropriate point at which to randomize before consent or after? Also, does consent to randomization adequately protect the interests of the individual subject? Or should the subject, in the name of autonomy or justice, be allowed to choose which arm or treatment s/he wants?[13]

3. Is the use of placebo as a control harmful and deceptive or necessary? Again, is consent to the possibility of placebo adequate to protect the individual's interests? If acceptable under some circumstances, are placebos unacceptable in life-threatening disorders? What are ethically and scientifically acceptable alternatives to the use of placebo (for example, other designs or other types of controls such as historical controls)?

4. When and under what conditions is it appropriate to communicate information obtained from the trial to the participants, to practicing clinicians, to the general public? How does one balance the need for firm evidence and valid and interpretable data with the desire and right of others to information? What information is "material" to subjects?

Many of the criticisms and challenges to clinical trial methodology expressed by the AIDS activists were not new, but had been debated by scientists and philosophers for years. What was new was the context, one of increased advocacy and empowerment of potential research subjects in the setting of an epidemic, which resulted in a reappraisal of the balance between protecting the rights and welfare of subjects and expanding their options for access to potentially beneficial but unproven drugs. This debate seems again to obscure the distinction between the goals of research and treatment, and highlights the reality that a significant portion of clinical research is performed with sick patients as subjects. Often these patients (and their physicians) have few other options and see participation in a clinical trial as a form of treatment. Even if "informed" that the benefit of the experimental therapy is unknown, most "consent" believing (at least in part) that it will help them.

THE RESPONSES

In response to the criticisms, both the FDA and the NIH altered the way they did business. Over the years, the FDA made dramatic philosophical and procedural changes in response to AIDS. All AIDS drugs have high priority for quick review. Under pressure from the activists, a rewrite of the IND regulations was issued in 1987 with the addition of a mechanism for a "treatment IND," and accelerated procedures in 1988. This was done in an effort to make drugs for serious or life-threatening diseases available faster, before a complete evaluation was done. The IND rewrite better defined the phases of clinical study and the criteria for review (Kessler). Phase I trials should generate sufficient safety data that a controlled Phase II trial can be designed to demonstrate that the drug works and what the common side effects are. Phase III goes on to establish the drug's effectiveness for specific indications and populations at risk. The new regulations limited the review of Phase I data to safety and the rights of the subjects, in an effort to reduce "regulatory impediments to scientific creativity" in the early stages of drug development (ibid.). Study design is reviewed only in Phase II and III research, with the FDA collaborating with the sponsor to ensure that the design is appropriate to ultimately obtain sufficient evidence of safety and efficacy for approval (Edgar and Rothman; Kessler; Mariner, 1990). By beginning review before the licensing application is complete, the FDA can cut months from the evaluation (Arno and Feiden, p. 238). The "treatment IND" regulations provided a new mechanism for the use of experimental (unapproved) drugs in life-threatening or serious diseases if no comparable or satisfactory treatment alternative is available. The drug must be under active investigation and must show some promise of therapeutic benefit (Edgar and Rothman; Kessler, p. 284; C. Levine, 1991a; Mariner, 1990; NRC). Since 1987, several drugs useful in the management of HIV have been available under a treatment IND, and a few of them have gone on to approval (C. Levine, 1991a).

The FDA has made two other major policy changes in response to criticisms and requests. The import policy, primarily in response to AIDS patients' requests for dextran sulfate, allows patients to import small quantities of an unapproved drug from foreign countries on a "pilot" basis in the absence of evidence of unreasonable risk or fraud (Annas, 1990; Kessler; C. Levine, 1991a; Mariner, 1990). Anyone can have access to any drug in the world, as long as it is for personal use only and a physician agrees to supervise its use (Edgar and Rothman; Kessler).

The other policy shift, partly a result of activist complaints that the 1987 regulation changes were too conservative, is the "parallel track" or expanded access program. Expanded and even earlier access to selected "promising" drugs is simultaneously available through a clinical trial and through the parallel track for those who are not eligible or able to participate in the clinical trial. After Phase I demonstration of reasonable safety with some prospect of efficacy, a drug could be obtained in parallel with the start of a Phase II trial. Expanded access requires that the manufacturer be willing to make adequate amounts of a drug available.[14] As of the end of 1992, three HIV antiviral drugs have been available through expanded access: dideoxyinosine (ddI), dideoxycytidine (ddC), and stavudine (D4T). All three have subsequently been approved. Ironically, although the drugs available through expanded access have been provided free by the sponsors, no consideration was given to the costs of associated laboratory monitoring and physician visits. This lack has led to the virtual exclusion of poor people from this program, despite the fact that the goal was increased access (C. Levine, 1991a; NRC)

With all of these changes, AIDS activists have succeeded in taking some of the decisions about risks and benefits of therapy out of the hands of the FDA staff and placing them in the hands of patients and nonresearch physicians (Edgar and Rothman, p. 137). At the same time, concern has been articulated about the impact of these changes on the clinical trials process and the possible sacrificing of the integrity of formal clinical trials. If drugs are widely available and assumed to be "effective" after Phase I trials (see Broder), how will we ever know if they are truly effective? Will Phase III clinical trials no longer be necessary? Will they even be possible because of the difficulties of recruitment and cost? Changes in drug regulation have occurred during the HIV epidemic, not because of public reaction to the tragic consequences of a drug or biologic as in the past, but because of strong consumer advocacy and activism leading a fight, often out of desperation, for earlier access to therapy. Whether any of these regulatory changes will affect the testing or licensing of HIV vaccines is unknown. Mariner (1990) argues persuasively that they should not because the majority of changes are specifically for drugs which *treat* life-threatening or serious diseases and therefore do not apply to vaccines which *prevent* disease.

Concurrent with changes in the regulatory process at the FDA, changes occurred at the NIH. The AIDS Clinical Trials Group (ACTG) of the National Institute of Allergy and Infectious Diseases (NIAID) had been created in 1986 as a national network of research sites prepared to conduct AIDS clinical trials. The ACTG had been slow to start, slow to recruit (resistant) patients, and accused of underincluding women and minorities. A restructuring of the system occurred in 1988; expansion was rapid, and an effort to enlist more and increasingly heterogeneous patients was being made. Activists called the ACTG "elitist," and controversy existed about whether research should be directed (activists' wish) or investigator-initiated (the traditional NIH approach); whether the research priority should be antiviral therapy (scientists' priority) or treatment of opportunistic diseases (activists' priority); and whether conflicts of interest (such as membership on the board of a company) influenced certain investigators' research (Arno and Feiden).

ACT-UP, already publicly critical of the clinical trials process, circulated a highly specific critique of the ACTG at the Fifth International AIDS Meeting in Montreal in 1989. Subsequently, an ACT-UP splinter group, the Treatment Action Group (TAG), has produced numerous documents suggesting changes in the clinical trials process and the ACTG. An NIAID scientist, Susan Ellenberg, organized an NIH-FDA conference on trial design, opening up a forum for discussion of novel trial designs as alternatives to the traditional randomized clinical trial by statisticians, clinical investigators, activists, and persons with AIDS. In late 1989, the ACTG awarded a new contract to the Statistical and Data Analysis Center at the Harvard School of Public Health, which formed a community advisory board to keep the community aware of activities and statistical issues. Some of the individual units (ACTUs) of the ACTG also formed community advisory boards. Now each ACTU is required to have a community advisory board to hear and address patient concerns and pertinent issues such as recruitment, retention, and compliance. By 1989–90 the NIAID Division of AIDS and the leadership of the ACTG included activists in many of their meetings. In July 1990, Dr. Anthony Fauci, director of NIAID, announced that activists would have representation on all committees and in all activities of the ACTG. The Community Constituency Group was established as a formal ACTG committee and continues to play an active and important role in the work of the ACTG.

Many clinical trials have relaxed their eligibility requirements to allow for the inclusion of more representative subjects. Most sites have made an effort to recruit underrepresented groups (for example, see Merrigan; Byar, 1990). Women have demanded participation in clinical trials for their own good, not just as mothers or "vectors" of transmission. Pediatric trials have, contrary to tradition and regulation, sometimes begun concurrently with adult trials (e.g., ddI).

The development of the Community Consortium of Bay Area HIV Providers, the Community Research Initiative (NYC 1987–1991), the NIAID Community Programs for Clinical Research in AIDS (CPCRA), and AmFAR's community research programs have created a large base of community-conducted clinical research in HIV, which is believed to have increased access, equity, and efficiency. These grassroots trials are seen as an important complement to research in traditional settings (Arno and Feiden, p. 123). Placebo controls are rarely used now in trials of HIV antiviral drugs because of the availability and effectiveness of AZT, setting this controversy aside at least temporarily. Activists, however, complain about the continued testing of AZT in clinical trials.

Perhaps the major change is that the entire clinical trials process is now open and highly visible. Many members of the public are familiar with the language and process of clinical trials and the names of several investigational drugs. "Promising" findings are often reported on television or in the print media after preclinical testing, and drugs are sometimes called "effective" after Phase I trials. Many worry that premature news coverage, sometimes claiming what sounds like success, may raise the expectations of the public and the affected community unfairly (Grodin, Kaminow, and Sassower). The extensive information network of the gay community allows widespread dissemination of information, misinformation, recipes, and rumors as soon as there are data with a hint of hope. "The public's perception that a drug is 'toxic' (and therefore worthy of dismissal) or 'effective' (and therefore worthy of wide-scale distribution) has become a common theme of Phase I drug development" (Broder, p. 418). The net result may be to impede the development of promising agents by making it difficult to complete the clinical trials process. Many believe that only proper clinical trials of experimental drugs will ultimately "relieve the most suffering and do the most good" (Richman, p. 413). Public presentation of data that are very early or inadequate and then change to reflect updated knowledge can lead to public alarm, confusion, and increased distrust of scientists, researchers, and the government. "Publicity of AIDS research has created a public image of medical research quite different from reality" (Grodin, Kaminow, and Sassower, p. 348).

Some studies may take longer to design because of input from various sources, but the final design may be more agreeable to participants and therefore enhance recruitment and compliance. While trials conducted with less strict eligibility criteria and more flexibility in the traditional methods may make clinical trial participation accessible to more people, they may also result in less firm or convincing evidence of a drug's safety and effectiveness compared to alternative treatments. Also, relaxed eligibility criteria usually mean that a larger sample is required; therefore more people may be exposed to unnecessary suffering. Uncontrolled studies might allow participants to all receive a "promising" agent and might even be able to prove the efficacy of a curative drug (which is unlikely in HIV), but they would not be able to demonstrate the effect of drugs (such as AZT or ddI) that help but do not cure, or unmask drugs that have more toxicity than efficacy (Richman, p. 413).

Although some have applauded many of the changes that have occurred as long overdue, others have warned of their impact on science and the ability to find firm answers regarding treatment, diagnosis, or prophylaxis (see Annas, 1990; Broder; Cooper; Edgar and Rothman; Freedman, 1992; Richman; Rothman and Edgar, 1992). An individual's perceived right to early access to unproven agents might impact negatively on the public or social benefit derived from determining which drugs are of net benefit and which are not (Annas, 1990; Cooper; Richman). Widespread, early access to unproven drugs, rather than being compassionate, may be harmful in several ways, including giving false hope to desperate patients; subjecting individuals to risks of harm with little or no benefit, and also to the loss of an opportunity to take something better; wasting resources, time, money, and hope on something of minimal or inconsequential value; delaying or preventing the documentation of benefit or proper use of a drug; impeding the drug development process and controlled studies because of difficulty in recruiting volunteers (who would want to take part in a clinical trial if he or she could get the drug without participating?) and of interpreting confusing data; and costing society money and delaying the licensure and availability of a more useful drug (Cooper; Richman; Stolley). Cooper, claiming that participation in a clinical trial is itself a benefit unavailable to people who get unproven drugs outside of established trials, says, "Enrollment in a clinical trial offers patients benefits regardless of their treatment group, in terms of more frequency and intensity of observation and care they receive during the study and the possibility of being first to receive the drug if it should prove better than the control" (p. 2445). Perhaps most convincing is the reality that ineffective or toxic drugs waste valuable financial resources, energies, and the hopes of thousands. Richman claims that for every ten HIV drug candidates, perhaps one is effective, one is toxic, and most are relatively safe and useless. "If a physician has 10 bottles of pills on his shelf, how will s/he know (without a clinical trial) which is the effective one?" (Richman, p. 414). Even less a desperate and vulnerable patient. Finding effective treatments for HIV requires carefully done science. However, this does not exclude as incompatible with good science increased flexibility and creativity with respect to methods, as well as accelerated review and attention by regulators.

In a stronger claim, Annas warns that changes generated by the fear of HIV and the hope for a scientific cure have "helped erode the distinction between experimentation and therapy," and have changed the major mission of the FDA from consumer protection to the promotion of medical technology (1990, p. 183). Consequently, people with AIDS, "already suffering from an incurable illness, [are put] at further risk of psychological, physical, and financial exploitation by those who would sell them useless drugs" (ibid., p. 184). In some respects, the pre-Kefauver amendment emphasis on safety as the critical criterion (almost regardless of efficacy) for making drugs available has made a comeback.

> However staunch the FDA defense of its prerogatives, the concessions it has already made—and will continue to make—will mean that consumers and doctors will be forced to make difficult decisions without substantive information at hand. There is bound to be more guesswork, more hunches, more variety, ultimately more "schools" of medicine—reminiscent of, but never quite duplicative of . . . the 19th century. It will be less feasible to define orthodoxy, more important for the patient and the physician to cite unimpeachable authority . . . finally, and with near certainty, the pendulum will swing again. (Edgar and Rothman, pp. 139–40).

Dramatic changes in the conduct of clinical trials and the regulation of new drugs, as described above, have been the result of HIV-related activism, community interest, and political pressure. When these changes are examined in light of the widely accepted principles and guidance articulated in the Belmont Report, several observations can be made.

1. The distinction between experimentation and therapy, as defined by the Belmont Report, has become blurred, or to some extent has been denied or eliminated.

2. The arguments and recommendations for changes in clinical research and regulation put forth by activists and their advocates are based on respect for autonomy as the dominant guiding principle, to be held prior to other principles:

• respect for the autonomy of the individual to choose the research or therapeutic risks s/he deems acceptable;

• respect for the autonomy of the individual to make his/her own choices rather than having regulators, scientists, or even physicians make them;

• increased availability of information, even preliminary information, as critical to making informed choices;

• autonomy as the basis for a perceived right to, and a resultant demand for, unproven drugs and participation in clinical research;

• respect for the autonomy and ability to make choices of groups of people currently protected as "vulnerable" by regulation.

3. Although beneficence/nonmaleficence are still very important, they are seen as secondary to autonomy, because of the claim that only individuals can define what is good and what is harmful for them. The role of beneficence is also cited as playing a role in obligating researchers and the funders of research *to do research* in order to improve medical care and promote and protect the health of the people.

4. Justice as a principle requiring equitable selection of subjects is still important, but equitable access is taken to mean making the opportunity to participate in research available to *anyone* who chooses to participate based on his or her own self-determination. If clinical research is perceived as health care and health care is perceived as a right, then justice demands that no one be denied access to both.

The history of the ethics of clinical research could be described as having gone through at least four broad and overlapping stages. In the first era there were few regulations, codes of ethics, or laws guiding researchers. Researchers, especially those who were also medical practitioners (and most were), were trusted to do the right thing. Peer censure was a critical means of minimizing fraud and abuse. There was little recognition of any difference between research and therapy, and in fact most therapy was "unproven" and in that sense experimental. Most research was done in an effort to treat and therefore hopefully benefit the individual subject. Many investigational therapies were dangerous or even fatal.

The second phase, beginning around World War II, was a "utilitarian" stage during which support of research expanded greatly and some centralization occurred. Researchers aimed to answer questions thought to be important to society, and in so doing they often "used" subjects who were considered available or unimportant. Participation in research was more of a burden than a benefit for the individual; the benefits accrued to other groups. Imposing this burden on subjects was justified by the importance of the questions to be answered. Subjects were making a contribution to society. There was a clear distinction between research and therapy, and nontherapeutic research was accepted as necessary for scientific and medical progress.

This second phase was followed by a lengthy and critical period of scientific and public concern and debate about the purposes, values, methods, and limits of human-subjects research. Accusations of abuse were abundant. Many struggled with the justification for, and limits of, doing human-subjects research. Scientists, medical organizations, and the public (through congressional commissions and other public forums) attempted to describe the purposes and limits of research.

This period of examination and definition was followed by a stage essentially of response to the "use" and abuse of subjects of research. It was an era during which regulations and social controls on research were established and codified in an effort to protect the welfare and rights of subjects. Research was still seen as a good for society, but it had to be done carefully, with substantial review, and with the risk to the individual never outweighing the benefit to the individual or to society. Careful risk/benefit assessment was and is required, and the importance of the question cannot justify excessive risk to the consenting subject. The informed consent of the subject became an essential component of any "ethical" research in order to protect the autonomy and interests of the individual. Independent review of all proposed research was required in order to check the possibility of misjudgment by an invested scientist. The goals of research and therapy were defined as clearly distinct, yet benefits to the individual can and often do result from both. The regulations and codes of ethics that we currently follow were all generated during this time.

Currently, we are perhaps in a new phase, at least with respect to perceptions and attitudes toward research. This phase might be described as one in which the *rights* of potential subjects are paramount and the demand for research is great. Research subjects have claimed a right to participate in research, a right to choose and make decisions, a right to take risks (as they define them), and a right to have access to experimental drugs. Although this is most pronounced among HIV-infected research subjects and their advocates, some similar claims are being made by persons with other diseases such as breast cancer and Alzheimer's disease. The benefits to subjects and to society of participating in biomedical research are emphasized, and the sense of "burden" is denied. The distinction between therapy and research is minimized. Participation in research is seen as a way (and for some is the only way) to obtain needed treatment and health care. It will be interesting to see how sustained this change of emphasis is, whether codes or regulations will change accordingly, and how and when the pendulum may swing again. Will the future of research ethics take a radically different course? If the ethics of clinical research at all parallels that of general medical ethics, it may be in the "midst of a profound transformation" (see, for example, Pellegrino, 1993).

THE ETHICS OF VACCINE RESEARCH

In all of the history and attention to the ethics of human-subjects participation in clinical research, the thinking and writing has concentrated primarily on the clinical investigation of new drugs for sick patients. "It has been assumed that guidelines and procedures for the regulation of clinical research applied also to research on biologicals. But in fact this is not so. Research on vaccines presents its own particular problems" (Mahler, p. xi). Historically, many of the first large clinical trials were trials of vaccines in large groups of people, yet there is remarkably little discussion or recognition of differences between the clinical investigation of drugs and of vaccines. As previously stated, the regulations governing the conduct of clinical trials for vaccines in the U.S. are the same as those for clinical trials of drugs.

Drugs are intended to treat an illness from which a person already suffers. Although the goal of a drug trial is not benefit for the individual but practical knowledge, the clinical investigation of a drug often results in direct and immediate benefit to the individual subject. The participant in a drug trial usually has the disease which the drug is intended to treat. Vaccines, on the other hand, are intended to *prevent* illness or infection in an individual as well as to protect others and the larger community. Vaccines are given to healthy individuals who might at some future time be exposed to the putative infection, but also may never be exposed. The participant in a vaccine trial, therefore, is asked to accept some element of risk now in exchange for a future personal benefit which may never be needed, and for the benefit of the community or society. One could argue that vaccine research qualifies neither as "medical research combined with professional care" (in which the aim is essentially diagnostic or therapeutic for the patient) nor as "nontherapeutic biomedical research" (the essential object of which is purely scientific and without implying direct diagnostic or therapeutic value to the subject) (Declaration of Helsinki), but really falls in some middle gray area. (See chapter 3 for more discussion of this point.) "Public health use of certain biologicals is clearly distinguishable from individual treatment . . . biologicals are preventive agents, employed for control of communicable disease, first by safeguarding individuals and, at the same time, protecting groups" (Ladimer, p. 111).

Since most vaccines to date are made of live-attenuated or killed microorganisms, healthy participants in vaccine trials may receive injections of potentially disease-causing pathogens. The proof of effectiveness of a vaccine is sometimes obtained by challenging the subjects under controlled conditions with unmodified pathogens. Preclinical evidence of vaccine safety and careful control of the conditions for challenge experiments minimize, but cannot eliminate, the risk inherent in these procedures (see chapter 1). Historically, populations used for early studies of vaccines included the institutionalized mentally impaired and prisoners, both because it was possible to control their environments and because infectious diseases were a common problem for these groups. Also frequently employed as subjects in vaccine experiments have been the investigators themselves (see Altman, 1987) and their families. Field studies of vaccines have often been done with children, primarily because they have been the population at most risk from vaccine-preventable infectious diseases. Since the work of the National Commission and subsequent regulations, the use of these groups (children, prisoners, the mentally impaired) as subjects in research has been greatly restricted.

In 1976 in Geneva, an "International Conference on the Role of the Individual and the Community in the Research, Development, and Use of Biologics," sponsored by the WHO, the CIOMS, the World Medical Association (author of the Declaration of Helsinki), the U.S. Centers for Disease Control (CDC), and the International Association of Biological Standardization, specifically addressed ethical issues particular to vaccine research. The proceedings of this conference offer a series of insightful discussions on vaccine research, development, and use, with attention to its unique aspects.

Of particular interest is the recommendation by several of the participants that vaccine research be recognized as "community research" (Crane; Ladimer) or "research in the public interest" (Dull and Bryan) in which the principal beneficiary is the public rather than the individual. Therefore a "complementary ethical foundation stressing societal as well as individual needs and benefits" is needed (Ladimer, p. 112). On this basis, a recommendation is made that the interests of the subject include and be consistent with the interests of each subject *as a member of the community*, thereby eliminating (or at least minimizing) conflict between the interests of the individual and the community. Some of the participants suggested that otherwise guidelines employed in the clinical investigation of therapeutics applied as well to that of preventive vaccines. The proceedings also contain "Criteria for Guidelines on the Role of the Individual and the Community in the Research, Development, and Use of Biologicals."

Most codes and guidelines of research ethics focus on research as therapeutic or nontherapeutic for the individual patient or participant, and not on research done for or with communities. The Nuremberg Code (1949) states: "The experiment should be such as to yield fruitful results for the good of society," recognizing that the research question must be of importance to more than the individual. The 1982 proposed CIOMS guidelines (following chronologically close behind the above-mentioned Geneva conference) specifically attempted to include community-based research. The stated purpose of these guidelines, in which the universal validity of the principles of the Declaration of Helsinki is recognized, is to suggest applicability of the principles to technologically developing countries, and to address "issues specific to research involving communities rather than individual subjects" (item 5). The CIOMS guidelines, while recognizing that in community-based research "individual consent on a person-to-person basis may not be feasible . . . and the decision to undertake the research will rest with the public health authority," state that "the ethical considerations and safeguards applied to research on individuals must be translated, in every possible respect, into the community context" (CIOMS, 1982, pp. 16 and 17).

CIOMS, again recognizing that existing codes did not adequately cover the special features of population-based or epidemiological studies, in 1991 issued proposed *International Guidelines for Ethical Review of Epidemiological Studies*.[15] The scope of these guidelines is broad, with the intention of covering all types of epidemiological research, including, as one example, large randomized trials of preventive vaccines.

In 1993, CIOMS, in response to advances in medical science and "new perceptions of what is ethical conduct" in research (including changes generated by the HIV epidemic), revised its 1982 guidelines with a goal of "striking a balance between the paramount ethical concern for vigilance in protecting the rights and welfare of research subjects and an ethical responsibility to advance the good of societies and of research subjects" through research (CIOMS, 1992 and 1993). In this document, respect for persons, beneficence, and justice are identified as the basic ethical principles which "guide the conscientious preparation of proposals for scientific studies," and these principles are applied to research involving human subjects.

CHAPTER THREE

▲
_____
▼

Human-Subjects Research
and HIV Vaccines

Rigorous evaluation of the safety and efficacy of vaccines requires clinical research with human subjects and raises important questions of ethics. Vaccines have been tested in human subjects many times over hundreds of years, and in many ways, both good and not so good by today's standards. Guidelines, regulations, and attitudes governing human-subjects research have evolved over time as scientific possibilities have expanded. Dull and Bryan note that the "process determining which biologicals came into being was a synthesis of what was *needed* to control or prevent important human diseases, what was *possible* in terms of existing scientific and technical knowledge, and what was *acceptable* with respect to relative value" (p. 118). Historically, as some infectious diseases have been conquered or controlled by effective vaccines and therapies, others have emerged to present new challenges. The need for biologicals is therefore always evolving. Scientific and technical knowledge has also continuously evolved. An explosion of scientific possibilities creating new strategies for vaccine development occurred with the advent of molecular biology and techniques of recombining DNA. Sociocultural attitudes toward vaccines and toward biomedical research, both basic and clinical, have evolved and changed as well. Some of the justifications and methods used to test vaccines in the past would no longer be permissible today. As described in the previous chapter, many of the national and international codes, laws, and regulations which are followed today were based on an assumption that medical research is hazardous to and exploitative of subjects. Hence, their main focus is protection of individual rights and welfare. Recently this basic assumption has been challenged by a growing perception (as articulated especially by HIV activists) that participation in research and access to investigational drugs is beneficial and therefore a right. Neither perception is entirely accurate, and the reality is probably somewhere in the middle (see, for example, R. Levine, 1993, p. 339).

Given the expected and desired societal benefit of having an HIV vaccine and the accepted process of conducting clinical trials to demonstrate vaccine safety and efficacy, this chapter will address whether and how clinical research with experimental HIV vaccines is justified and under what conditions. First the goal of and justification for human-subjects research will be examined, with a review of the usual interpretation of ethical principles accepted as foundational for the conduct of human-subjects research. It will then be argued that (1) research and clinical trials of vaccines are significantly different from clinical research of drugs or therapeutics; (2) because of these differences, vaccine research (including but not limited to HIV) falls outside of the two categories of research (clinical or therapeutic and nonclinical or nontherapeutic) identified by the Declaration of Helsinki; and (3) also because of these differences, vaccine research may not comply with a strict (but common) interpretation of ethical guidance available through existing codes and regulations for human-subjects research. Thus a third legitimate category of research should perhaps be added, based on an understanding of research designed to benefit the community, and a slightly expanded interpretation of the ethical principles relevant to and foundational for human-subjects research.

Research is an activity aimed at advancing practical knowledge toward the improvement of medical care and the public health. The "client" of research includes society at large and future generations, but also the immediate beneficiaries of any experimental intervention proved to be useful. Beneficiaries may be individual participants, groups with which an individual identifies (communities), or society. Current ethical guidance recognizes only two of these, individuals and society. Research whose goal is the improvement of the public health, and this includes vaccine research, targets the community as the primary beneficiary.

DIFFERENCES BETWEEN VACCINE RESEARCH AND DRUG RESEARCH

There is remarkably little discussion in the literature of the substantial differences between clinical trials of drugs or therapeutics and clinical trials of vaccines.[16] The main differences pertain to the composition and size of the sample and to whom benefits primarily accrue. Because vaccine research involves large numbers of healthy persons and intends to benefit the community as much as or more than each individual, analysis of risks and benefits for vaccine research must be different from that for drug research.

Subjects recruited for participation in clinical trials of drugs, at least at the stage of establishing and confirming efficacy, almost always have the disease the drug is designed to treat. Despite the concerns of some that illness makes them vulnerable to undue influences, subjects are nevertheless patients in need of treatment, and the experimental treatment, although of uncertain effectiveness, is perhaps one of very few options which could benefit them directly.[17] Subjects in therapeutic studies are willing to accept some risk and uncertainty for the possibility of a direct and immediate benefit which they are in need of now. Because an effect (or lack of one) will be seen in each subject, the number of subjects needed is relatively small. Finding an effective therapy has potential immediate benefit for the individual with the given disease, and potential future benefit for the group of individuals who have the disease, and for society at large because of the advancement of useful knowledge.

On the other hand, subjects recruited for participation in clinical trials of vaccines are *healthy* individuals who *may at some future time* be at risk from the disease which the vaccine is designed to prevent. It is also possible that they will never be exposed to, or infected with, the putative agent, or that it could occur many years later. "In vaccine trials there are no patients, in that only a small number of vaccinees will ever become victims of the disease even if no effective vaccine is given" (Bjune and Gedde-Dahl, p. 2). Because an effect will be seen in only a small portion of vaccinated individuals anyway, large numbers of participants are needed. All participants are at risk from the side effects of the vaccine, but only some are at risk from the infectious disease, and for those it is a future risk. There may, however, be a psychological benefit in feeling "protected," especially if the risk of infection is spread fairly evenly. Therefore there is limited immediate benefit to the individual, and future benefit only to some. Vaccination of individuals also serves to reduce the reservoir for, and therefore transmission of, infection in the community. So subjects in vaccine research accept some risk and uncertainty for the possibility of a potential future benefit which they may never need, for the more immediate benefit of the community by reducing risk and disease, and for the advancement of usable knowledge.

COMMUNITY AS THE PRIMARY BENEFICIARY OF VACCINE RESEARCH

In addition to the production of knowledge, the possible decrease in morbidity and mortality associated with a given disease, and the possible restoration of health (and productivity) of some of its members, the community is a beneficiary of vaccine research and utilization in an additional and perhaps more direct way: Through herd immunity, the risk to unvaccinated members of the community of contracting an infectious disease is reduced if a sufficient number of people are vaccinated. Although some vaccines are more effective in establishing herd immunity than others, one of the acknowledged goals of any vaccination program is to vaccinate a sufficient percentage of the community that the availability and the transmission of the infectious agent are reduced. If the vaccine is effective in reducing transmission and the incidence of the disease in the community, some risk to, and lack of protection for, the individual may be tolerated.[18] Vaccine research, although its purpose, like that of all research, is to generate usable knowledge in the service of health care, can potentially provide direct benefit, first to the community, and secondarily to the individual. Individuals benefit indirectly as members of the community, and a small percentage of them may benefit directly in the future.

Dull and Bryan suggest that at some point in history, "biologicals research and development became a 'public interest' responsibility" (p. 121). Biologicals came to be understood as essential for ensuring the health of the public as part of, and in addition to, ensuring the health of individuals. If, as they argue, biologicals are "public goods," i.e., goods enjoyed by all and involving government expenditures on behalf of the public, then biologicals research is done on behalf of the public and should be recognized as "research in the public interest." This would distinguish it from research "oriented toward personal health goals like disease therapy in which the public at large can expect little collective benefit" (ibid., p. 123). Dull and Bryan define research in the public interest as "that part of the total research effort of which the principal beneficiary is the public, not the individual, and thereby, in which the public has a special duty to encourage, financially support, and participate" (ibid.). A legitimate category of research should be recognized in which the primary beneficiary is the community or group of people with whom individuals identify.

The differences described above suggest that the risk-benefit analysis for vaccine research is different from that for drugs. Vaccines are "unavoidably unsafe," given to healthy persons not to treat them but to offer insurance against potential future infection. The more members of the community that are "insured," the better for the community. The risk or "premium" paid by the individual is exposure to mild or infrequent (albeit sometimes severe) side effects, and other inconveniences in the interests of the community and its members. For these reasons, an assessment of the potential risks and benefits of vaccine research to the community should always form an important part of its justification.

THE GOAL OF RESEARCH
AND WHO BENEFITS

Research has been defined as an activity "designed to test an hypothesis, permit conclusions to be drawn, and thereby to develop or contribute to generalizable knowledge" (National Commission, 1979, p. 3), as distinguished from practice, which refers to "interventions that are designed solely to enhance the well-being of an individual patient (or group) . . . and have a reasonable expectation of success" (ibid.). The primary justification for doing research is social beneficence. The social benefits to be gained thereby are substantial, and the risks of not doing research potentially great. Biomedical research in particular is necessary in order to know how to benefit patients through the practice of medicine. "It is very difficult to know truly in medicine; and since medical knowledge is knowledge in the service of action, false knowledge can lead to well-intentioned interventions causing patients needless harm" (Engelhardt, 1988, p. 124). Research is instrumental not only to the goods and goals of medicine (in which the individual is the primary focus of concern) but also to the goods and goals of public health (in which communities and the public are the focus of concern). Since medical practice concentrates on the well-being of human beings, research designed to improve medical practice must involve human beings as subjects. In the same way, research designed to improve the public health, whose focus is the health and well-being of communities, must involve communities as subjects.

The practice of human experimentation for the purpose of developing practical knowledge is *prima facie* good. "It is good and appropriate to encourage research with human subjects where such can lead to a better understanding of what will serve as efficacious treatment (including preventive medicine)" (ibid., p. 125); i.e., research is necessary for good medicine and public health. Some have suggested that there is a responsibility or an obligation to do research as "one means of improving medical care and protecting the health of the people" (CIOMS, 1992, p. 4). If research is considered a good or an obligation for the benefit of the people, the role of the research subject is not that of a "thing coopted into the service of alien goals, exploited by those who want to pursue scientific progress, but, rather of an individual cooperating in an important social goal of importance to that individual as well" (Engelhardt, 1986, p. 292).

Recent interest in revisiting the ethics of clinical research has been generated in part by an evolving appreciation of the value of clinical research, which has been manifested by some as a demand for research. "Concern for the protection of human subjects cannot justify what might be regarded as the ethically neutral stance of avoiding or refraining from research involving human subjects. When biomedical research involving human subjects is seen as beneficial and ethically proper rather than only as exposure to risk, research subjects must be regarded as beneficiaries of research and not only as possible victims" (CIOMS, 1992, p. 4). This statement reflects the perception of some that participation in biomedical research is an opportunity, or even a benefit to which they are entitled, rather than a burden from which they must be protected. This view, along with advances in biomedical science which expand the potential for human biomedical research, the influence of the HIV epidemic, and the increasing volume of international research, has created an impetus for a reexamination of the ethics of clinical research (see also chapter 2). Interestingly, the final version of the CIOMS 1993 *International Ethical Guidelines for Biomedical Research Involving Human Subjects* recognizes this view that participation in research can be a benefit and attributes it largely to the influence of the HIV epidemic. However, this recognition is accompanied by a strong sense of caution: "Many people regard this claim with apprehension in case research will be undertaken or promoted without adequate justification and secure safeguards of the rights and welfare of the research subjects" (CIOMS, 1993, p. 9).

Whatever the extent of change in perception about the personal benefits of participation in research, tension between the interests of the individual and those of society is presumed to exist. Rather than recognizing a need for social controls to prevent scientists and society from "exposing persons to harm" by "using" them as subjects of research, some individuals are insisting that such controls are paternalistic and restrictive, are "demanding" that research be done, and are "demanding" to participate because it is beneficial to them. Alternatively, it could be suggested that a basis of tension between the interests of the individual and those of the community or society is not necessary. If community, societal, and individual interests are related and not at odds, individuals who participate in research can perceive themselves as participants in an effort to solve an important community problem. Researchers are also participants in this endeavor and therefore will undertake only research that is adequately justified and respectful of the rights and welfare of all participants.

THE BELMONT PRINCIPLES

In the Belmont Report (1979), the National Commission identified and described three fundamental ethical principles as particularly relevant to the ethics of research involving human subjects: respect for persons, beneficence, and justice (these are described in chapter 2). The CIOMS, in both its 1982 and 1993 guidelines, embraces the same three principles as providing guidance for the conduct of human-subjects research. However, given the accepted interpretations of these principles, justification of certain kinds of research, of which vaccine research is one example, is problematic, as is reconciling inevitable conflicts between the principles.

Marshall argues that autonomy and justice are deontological principles "which single out the research subject as the focus of moral concern . . . the person whose rights and welfare are paramount" (p. 5). The principle of beneficence and the related requirement for risk/benefit assessment are different. Here, the welfare of the subject is *not* the sole interest, because research is not intended to benefit the research subject, and in fact it may be detrimental to his/her welfare. Beneficence is a "utilitarian principle . . . which seeks the good of some aggregate of which the research subject is at best merely a part" (ibid.). Marshall contends that the balancing of principles is very difficult because they are based on different types of ethical considerations. He suggests that respect for persons and justice should always outweigh "benefits" to society in review by the institutional review board (ibid., p. 6).

Veatch argues that beneficence (social and/or individual) is the minimally necessary condition for ethically acceptable research (1987, p. 28), but that considerations of benefit and harm come into play only when other conditions, particularly those protecting the rights of subjects, are met. The nonconsequentialist principles, autonomy and justice, always take priority—i.e., they must be satisfied before the consequences are considered—and beneficence can never justify their being compromised (ibid., pp. 28, 45).

Since the primary argument for doing human-subjects research is social beneficence, research contributing to generalizable knowledge must be guided by questions designed to improve medical care or the public health. Therefore, the most fundamental question to be addressed in justifying research with human subjects as ethical is "Will the answer to this scientific question potentially benefit people?" By itself, however, that is not enough. The scientific quest for improvement in medical practice or public health must be limited by respect for those participating in the research and by equity in sharing the benefits and burdens. Respect for participants need not be limited, however, to respect for the autonomy rights of individuals. Respect may also be warranted because of other aspects of being a person.[19] Communities of persons should be afforded respect as well and acted toward benevolently. Balancing protection of individual autonomy and just treatment of the individual with benefit to others is not straightforward. Yet, regulations and available guidance suggest that these principles must be satisfied without specifying how to balance them, or which should take priority. Balancing benefit to a community of persons with whom the individual identifies with respecting each individual member of that community (for more than his/her ability to be autonomous) and treating each member equitably may be easier to achieve and is a reasonable application of the three principles to vaccine research.

A partnership between the investigators, the community, and the members of the community should be the basis for the conduct of vaccine research. Robert Veatch (1987) suggests a partnership between research subject and researcher, one in which the overlap of interests, the point at which there might be mutual interests, is found. However, it may not always be true that the interests of the researcher (or the subject) represent the interests of society. When individuals are understood as communal and it is recognized that the individual good and the common good can be inextricably interrelated, the presumed tension between individual and societal interests in the conduct of research fades. A community can be thought of as composed of and representing its members, so that what is defined and recognized by the members as good for the community of which the individual is a member is good for the individual, and is therefore worth some cost. Well-done research conducted to answer a question which is of importance to the members of a community is good for the community. Yet there has been little recognition in the literature that the value of research to the community also promotes the interests of the individual as a *member* of that community. Conceived of in this way, the subject is not merely a means to an end or a passive participant in research and in need of protection, but an active participant in agreeing to the ends themselves and to the means of reaching them. The issue of social justice is also addressed because the burdens of research are primarily shouldered by the same group as the benefits.

Respect for Persons
Current guidance describes respect for persons as principally respect for the self-determined choices of autonomous individuals, i.e., those capable of deliberation about personal choices (National Commission, 1979, p. 4).[20] As autonomous agents, individuals may consent to participate in research even if it entails some risk to them. Current guidance, however, also includes an element of protecting even autonomous individuals from choosing inordinate or unjustified (by corresponding benefits) risks, since research presented to autonomous individuals must first satisfy the IRB that benefits outweigh risks.

Dr. Robert Levine notes that "to show respect for autonomous persons requires that we leave them alone, allowing them to choose their own activities . . . we are not to touch them or encroach on their space unless . . . [it] is in accord with their wishes" (1986, p. 16). The principle of respect for persons in the context of ethical guidance for human-subjects research is often referred to and understood as respect for autonomy. Levine argues that respecting autonomy requires that our actions be designed to affirm individuals' authority and enhance their capacity to be self-determining.

Respect for persons entails more, however, than just leaving people alone to make their own choices, and more than just respect for their autonomy (as beneficence entails more than just not harming people). A person is more than merely an individual bearer of rights. If it is only autonomy that deserves respect, then for what reason should nonautonomous individuals such as children or the mentally incompetent be protected and respected? And yet, this is the second conviction espoused by the National Commission under the auspices of respect for persons (1979, p. 4). We should respect persons as living human beings with multiple capacities, including who they are and how they make choices. That may require that our actions be designed to affirm their wholeness and enhance different human capacities in addition to the capacity to be self-determining. Respecting persons also implies not harming them (nonmaleficence), as well as protecting them from inordinate or unjustified harm, and maybe even promoting their interests (beneficence). In the case of research, respect for persons should include respecting their communal or social nature and enhancing their capacity to be public-spirited rather than solely self-interested.

The National Commission and most available codes of research ethics have adopted an "atomistic view of the person" as "a highly individualistic bearer of rights and duties; among his or her rights, some of the most important are to be left alone, not to be harmed, and to be treated with fairness" (R. Levine, 1986, p. 13). This perception, which dominates research ethics, is understandable because it was adopted in the 1970s in response to prior abuse of persons as research subjects and the assumption that being a research subject was a burden. This view also reflects the basic values of a liberal political philosophy. However, it does not reflect the richness of being a person and the perception of persons as social beings with a stake in social goals. Instead of individualism, a view of persons as beings who exist in relation to others and whose very being is in part defined by these relationships may be more appropriate as a basis for describing respect for persons in the context of research, and probably in other contexts as well. By supplementing (but not replacing) basic liberal values (such as liberty and justice) with communitarian values (such as community, caring, and solidarity), respect for persons could include respect for an individual's relatedness to others, for the obligations and interests that this relatedness entails, and for individuals' potential to be public-spirited and in solidarity with others and with their communities.[21] Respect for persons should also include respect for the communities to which these individuals belong. Respect for the community could be justified as an extension of personal autonomy rights, i.e., community autonomy or the right of a group of individuals to collectively determine their group's action (see S. Hall, 1992). It could also include respect for the well-being of the community as composed of members with common interests and a common good. As Larry Gostin notes: "The importance of group identity, and of treating social communities with dignity and respect, is increasingly well-recognized" (1991, p. 192).

Justice
The principle of justice as applied to the conduct of human-subjects research requires a fair distribution of the benefits and burdens of research. The principle of justice in codes and regulations of research ethics has been applied primarily to the equitable selection of subjects and the fair distribution of burdens and benefits, including results (or resulting benefits). Expanding respect for persons beyond respect for autonomy, and understanding beneficence as pertaining to individuals, groups, and society at large do not change the implied requirements of applying the principle of justice. Individual research subjects *and* groups or communities of subjects must be selected for reasons related to the problem(s) to be studied and the potential of benefit, and not because of convenience, manipulability, or other nonrelevant differences. Individuals and communities participating in research should be selected because they are its potential beneficiaries and because they understand and have voluntarily consented to take part. The risks of research designed to benefit many people should be spread fairly. Individuals and communities that participate in research, and thereby accept the risks and burdens, should be ensured of sharing in the resulting benefits. Justice should also be appealed to in decisions about what research should be done and how research dollars should be allocated.

Beneficence
The principle of beneficence is described as including two complementary rules: (1) do no harm, and (2) maximize possible benefits and minimize possible harms (National Commission, 1979, p. 4). The commission interpreted beneficence as creating an obligation to secure the well-being of

individuals and to develop information that will form the basis of our being better able to do so in the future. This interpretation and its application in codes and regulations of research ethics affirm the goal of social beneficence forwarded by the conduct of useful and well-designed research. A major limiting factor expressed by the principle of beneficence is that subjects must not be intentionally harmed or injured (nonmaleficence toward individuals always takes precedence over beneficence to society).[22] How to assess risks and benefits, and how to balance risks and benefits to society with those to individuals or groups of individuals participating in research, is a complex issue.

If an important general justification of human-subjects research is social beneficence, it has been presumed that the interests of the individual are then at risk and must be protected from being "used" by society for society's ends. Many have struggled with the ethical tension between the interests of the individual and those of society:

> When science takes man as its object, tensions arise between two values basic to Western society: freedom of scientific inquiry and protection of individual inviolability. Both are facets of man's quest to order his world. Scientific research has given man some, albeit incomplete, knowledge and tools to tame his environment while commitment to individual worth and autonomy, however wavering, has limited man's intrusions on man. Yet, when human beings become the subject of experimentation, allegiance to one value invites neglect of the other. At the heart of this conflict lies an age-old question: When may society, actively or by acquiescence expose some of its members to harm in order to seek benefits for them, for others, or for society as a whole? (Katz, Capron, and Glass, p. 1)

Human-subjects research, even though done in pursuit of knowledge to improve medical practice or the public health, has often been narrowly understood as "society exposing its members to harm." The conflict most consistently invoked in the literature is the polarity of individual good and the common good, between private and public welfare. Hans Jonas (1970) developed this conflict eloquently, describing "conscription" of subjects to "sacrifice" themselves in the service of the "collective." However, Jonas also denies the social good inherent in clinical research and suggests instead that scientific progress is optional.

Protection of the rights, interests, and well-being of the individual as the main consideration in ethical guidance concerning the conduct of clinical research has been criticized by international scientists, representatives of developing countries, epidemiologists, and others. Some have argued stridently for a better balance between individual interests and society's interests (Ackerman, 1992; Eisenberg, 1977; R. Levine, 1993). Some critics have claimed that the research codes' emphasis on individualism and protection of individual rights (based on a Western political liberal philosophy) is incompatible with less individualistic cultural and moral perspectives in which persons define themselves in relation to their community, and in which conflict between the interests of the individual and the community would be hard to imagine (Ajayi; Barry; La Vertu and Linares; R. Levine, 1982; J. Miller; and others).[23]

Epidemiologists have also been critical: "A person dominated medical ethic . . . that focuses primarily on individual rights and duties and does not see individuals as part of a wider social order and community is insufficient for the task of setting moral and human rights boundaries around the conduct of research on populations" (Gostin, 1991, p. 191). The development of the CIOMS *International Guidelines for the Review of Epidemiological Studies* (1991) was an attempt to recognize the unique aspects of epidemiological research, that which "concerns groups of people." Emphasis is placed on potential benefits and harms to the group or culture being studied. These guidelines describe epidemiological research as including both observational and experimental studies, and cite large-scale vaccine research as an example of an experimental study. What is left unclear is whether those conducting vaccine research are supposed to adhere to these guidelines or to the CIOMS *International Ethical Guidelines for Biomedical Research Involving Human Subjects* (CIOMS, 1993) (or both?). If the distinction is that biomedical research involves primarily individuals and epidemiological research involves primarily communities, then it could be argued that vaccine research is both. Vaccine research involves applying an intervention to individuals which entails risk and benefit to the individual and risk and benefit to the community, for the benefit of the health of the community and its members.

Smith and Morrow suggest that the appropriate balance in research between benefit for the individual and benefit for society at large depends on the particular situation. They argue that "resolution depends on where investigators place their horizon of responsibility"—confined to the study participants or extended to the entire population to which the intervention may sometime be applied (p. 72). In reality, investigators do not have this choice but have a responsibility to both. They are ethically obligated to design and conduct valid research that will generate knowledge that is beneficial to society (useful at least for the population to which the intervention will be applied), *and* they are obligated to protect the rights and welfare of individuals who participate in the conduct of such research. The horizon of responsibility is fluid only to the extent that individual participants are benefited, and this should be defined by the type and phase of research and the interests of the subjects and the community rather than investigator discretion. Ambiguous and sometimes vague regarding balance, codes of research ethics emphasize the responsibility of the investigator to the individual study participants (primarily as a check to scientific ambition or a utilitarian justification for research), failing to recognize that some research has no potential direct benefit for the individual participant.

Veatch suggests an alternative rather than having to choose between the interests of society and those of the individual. His model is a partnership between the researcher and the subject, "a convergence or mutuality of interests" where "both have something to gain and each is called upon to make some sacrifice for the benefit of the other" (1987, p. 5). As described above, the idea of research as a partnership can be viewed as the most appropriate foundation for the ethics of research, in which investigators and subjects are "partners" in pursuit of an answer to a socially important question. In the case of vaccine research (or other research that fits into the same category, as defined below), the partnership is really a three-way partnership between the community, individual members of the community, and the investigator(s). "If the researcher and the subject [community] are seen as partners who are both [all] autonomous, responsible, dignified human agents [or groups of human agents] coming together to form a limited covenant for pursuit of a mutual interest, virtually all aspects of the ethics of clinical research are affected. It provides a new foundation for ethically acceptable clinical research" (ibid., p. 4).

INADEQUACIES OF AVAILABLE GUIDANCE

Available guidance found in codes of research ethics and regulations governing human-subjects research can be seen as conflicting or too vague to be helpful in reconciling the presumed conflict between the interests of society and those of the individual, especially with respect to research which benefits society but may not have direct benefit for the individual subject.

Declaration of Helsinki
The Declaration of Helsinki recognizes that in some biomedical research (nonclinical or nontherapeutic), the "essential object . . . is purely scientific and without implying direct diagnostic or therapeutic value to the persons subjected to the research" (Introduction). However, one of the Declaration's basic principles, that "concerns for the interests of the subject must always prevail over the interests of science and society" (I.5), and another statement, that "in research on man, the interests of science and society should never take precedence over considerations related to the well-being of the subject" (III.4), appear to contradict the defined goal of nontherapeutic or nonclinical research. If the aim of nonclinical research is purely scientific, then the interests of science *do* take precedence over the interests of the subject. The goal is scientific knowledge acquired by exposing the subject to at least some risk without direct benefit. Likewise, if the aim of nonclinical research is the good of society, then the interests of society take precedence over those of the subject. Individuals do not participate in "nontherapeutic" research for their own benefit or in their own interests unless their interests include concern for the welfare of others or for a group. Strict interpretation of statements from the Declaration of Helsinki would make research which involved risk to the subjects, with no direct benefit (even if it is beneficial to society or a group of people), unethical according to the principles set forth.

Categories of Research

Human-subjects research to determine the efficacy of vaccines is neither "clinical (therapeutic)" nor "nonclinical (nontherapeutic)" as distinguished by the widely accepted Declaration of Helsinki. "In the field of biomedical research a fundamental distinction must be recognized between medical research in which the aim is essentially diagnostic or therapeutic for a patient ('clinical'), and medical research the object of which is purely scientific and without implying direct diagnostic or therapeutic value to persons subjected to research ('non-clinical')" (Introduction). Although Phase I and II vaccine research, especially if carried out on low-risk populations, fits the description of nontherapeutic research, Phase III is more problematic. Some have argued that because the subjects of Phase III vaccine research include persons at risk of infection and likely target groups of an effective vaccination, they *do* stand to benefit from the research (Kostrzewski; Ladimer).[24] Others argue that vaccine trials are nontherapeutic because any individual benefit is marginal and uncertain at best (Bjune and Gedde-Dahl). Vaccine trials do not use a "new diagnostic or therapeutic measure" that offers "hope of saving life, reestablishing health or alleviating suffering" (therapeutic or clinical research), nor are they the "purely scientific application of medical research carried out on a human being" (nonclinical biomedical research), and therefore vaccine trials do not fit into either of the Helsinki categories. The recent CIOMS guidelines (1993), although claiming that administration of a vaccine is intended to be a benefit to the subject, agree with this interpretation: "Phase III vaccine trials do not conform to either of the categories defined in the Declaration of Helsinki" (Annex 2, p. 52).

However, these guidelines do not offer a resolution to this stated problem. A third category of research should be recognized. The Helsinki distinction is based on an analysis of benefit to individual subjects. Engelhardt (1988) suggests that there are actually *three* genres of human experimentation according to who the primary beneficiary is: (1) those with possible direct benefit for the patient-subject (such as Helsinki's "clinical"); (2) those likely to be of direct benefit to a class of individuals with which the subject identifies (in the sense of seeking the good of this class); and (3) those that bear no fruit of direct benefit to the subject (such as Helsinki's "nonclinical"). The acknowledgment and addition of a distinct category of research similar to Engelhardt's second would provide a fit for Phase III vaccine trials. This category would include all research in which the aim is essentially benefit to a group or community rather than (or in addition to) the health of individuals. Research falling into this category would define investigators' "horizon of responsibility" as primarily extending to the group or community which may directly benefit, yet still including responsibility for the interests and rights of individual subjects, and an obligation to design and conduct research which will provide a valid contribution (benefit) to society. Vaccine research is likely to be of direct benefit to a class of individuals to which an individual subject belongs, that class usually being a group at particular risk from the infectious disease (which in the case of HIV could be defined geographically or behaviorally). Benefits will also accrue to the community or society at large. If a third category of research were added to the Declaration of Helsinki with the stated aim of "benefit to the class of individuals with which the subject identifies," the interests of the class or community and the interests of its individuals would be compatible, and both would potentially be served by the conduct of such research. Obligations of justice would also be served, because individual subjects would always be recruited from groups that would likely benefit from the application of the investigational intervention.

Federal Regulations Governing Human-Subjects Research

Current U.S. regulations governing the conduct of human-subjects research (U.S. 45CFR.46) are also not particularly helpful in reconciling presumed conflicts between benefits to individuals and benefits to society. Regulations instruct IRBs to review research to determine such things as whether "risks to subjects are reasonable in relation to benefits, if any, to the subject and the importance of the knowledge that may reasonably be expected to result" (45CFR.46.III(2)). Yet nowhere do the regulations define what is "reasonable" with respect to risk (only "minimal risk" is defined), especially in relation to studies with a remote possibility of benefit to the subject. Nor, and perhaps more important, is it clear how or by whom the importance of the expected knowledge is to be determined. Veatch (1987) suggests that risk/benefit evaluations and evaluation of the importance of the sought-after knowledge are very subjective and therefore should be made by the individual research subject. In the model proposed in this book, the community in which an effective vaccine would be utilized and from which individual participants in the research would be recruited and selected would decide how important the expected knowledge is to them as a group, and how much risk and burden they are willing to accept in order to obtain this knowledge. This could be accomplished through a series of town meetings or public forums between investigators and members of the community for which an effective vaccine is intended. These meetings not only would serve to evaluate the potential risks and benefits of vaccine research and the importance of the knowledge to be gained as defined by that community, but could also serve to begin the process of informing potential participants, and allow for their input into the design and methods with which they would be willing to cooperate and comply. When an IRB subsequently reviews the ethics of the proposed research, it should have access to deliberations and conclusions reached by the community.

An additional difficulty with the current U.S. regulations is the instruction that "the IRB should not consider possible long-range effects of applying knowledge gained in the research as among those research risks that fall within the purview of its responsibility" (45CFR.46.111 (a)(2)). If the goal of research is social benefit, both the short- and long-term benefits and risks of the process and outcomes of research should be considered before it is initiated and are important considerations in determining whether vaccine research should be conducted. Consideration of only short-term risks, and only to the subject, in comparison to short- and long-term benefits to both the subject and society inevitably skews the balance in favor of benefits. If the IRB does not consider the possible long-term negative consequences of research, then someone else must. Both types of risks and benefits for participants and potential beneficiaries of research should be considered by a number of reviewers, including initially a national research priority-setting body (if one exists) and ethical review groups at the national and international level, but also by the communities deliberating about participation in research, by the IRBs which review the specific research proposals, and by individuals deciding whether or not to participate.[25] The IRB's consideration of long-term risks and benefits may be focused on the defined class of research subjects rather than just individuals. Dubler and Sidel suggest that even the restrictive formula for assessing risks found in the current regulations does not clearly "preclude weighing risks to a defined class of subjects, assuming the IRB has established the appropriateness of its jurisdiction over these matters" (p. 193).

The origin and intent of the research code statements and regulations cited above are understandable in a historical context of abuse of research subjects (see chapter 2) and justifiable in the light of limits on socially beneficent research based on risk of harm to the individual. Nonetheless, strict interpretation of these statements may make some research which is now conducted (for example, Phase III vaccine research) noncompliant and suspect, and also may limit the possibility of certain kinds of research.[26] Research which entails some risk to the individual without at least the intention of resulting in direct benefit to the individual is done in the interests of science and society, with the prospect of benefit to future persons or groups of persons (which may include the individual subject). Such research does place the interests of society or a group over those of the individual subject, while available guidance seems to suggest that this is not acceptable. Research of which the primary potential beneficiary is a community of persons should be recognized as legitimate. Justification of such research requires an evaluation by the community of benefits and risks to the community as well as to involved individuals. If persons identify themselves as members of the community and ascribe to the goals and interests of the community, and if the benefits of research to the community are recognized by its members as important and achievable, then clinical research that presents some risk without direct benefit to the individual is acceptable, and in some cases perhaps even necessary. The "horizon of responsibility" of the involved investigators then includes the community which has consented to the research and for which the application of the intervention will be a benefit. This is not to ignore history and the need to protect individuals from abuse, nor is it a utilitarian argument (justifying potential harm to the individual for the greater good of the aggregate), but rather a suggestion that balance can be achieved between a triad of interests: those of scientists and the scientific process, those representing the inviolability and dignity of individuals, and those that are valuable or good for the community or the common interest. This balance can be achieved by viewing the community of individuals which can benefit from the research as the "subject of research" and as a partner in the research enterprise. The three-way partnership allows for a convergence and mutual satisfaction of the interests of the community, the individual members of the community, and the scientists involved. Just as Veatch suggested for the researcher/subject partnership, the "result is a radically different and new moral basis" for research ethics (1987, p. 4).

When conducting research of this type, investigators will have responsibilities to the community (they have no such responsibility when conducting "therapeutic" research with individuals). Investigators and reviewers will be required to consider short- and long-term benefits and risks to communities involved in this category of research (community beneficence). Investigators are responsible for approaching target communities to present their proposal to them in order to inform the community; obtain the community's evaluation of the inherent risks and benefits; obtain the community's informed consent; and negotiate with the community about the specifics of the research design and associated commitments, before recruiting individual subjects for participation (respect for community autonomy). Within the consenting community, justice or fairness in the selection of potential participants must be adhered to. This means equity in the opportunity to participate as well as no coercion or manipulation. Consideration must also be given to social justice, i.e., ensuring that the community will be able to participate in the benefits of the research.

In the case of HIV vaccine research, the specific end is prevention of a disease which is devastating to the community or society in which the individual lives and/or with which he or she identifies. Human-subjects research conducted in pursuit of a vaccine to prevent HIV is valuable to the community, and therefore to individuals as members of the community.

COMMUNITY

The concept of "community" is complex, has been variously defined, and is loosely used. Key concepts generic to all definitions are that a community is a group or aggregate of people who interact with each other, are interdependent, and have something in common (whether it be ancestry, place of inhabitancy, culture, behaviors, or special interests), and who understand or define themselves to some extent as belonging to this group.

Three general types or categories of community have been described: structural, emotional, and functional (Archer). Structural communities are aggregates of people who are gathered for a variety of reasons. Included are face-to-face communities (such as neighborhoods, tribes, families), geopolitical communities, organizations (e.g., churches, health departments, labor unions), special-risk communities (e.g., those at high risk for a certain disease), and others (Archer; Blum). Emotional communities center around a sense or feeling of community, "a place where one belongs . . . a place where an individual is known . . . and safe to be known" (Keyes, p. 14); they may be created around a common set of transient or long-term special interests (Blum, p. 501). Functional communities are those that, based on some sense of common need, interest, or problem, function as a community to try to solve a problem or fill a need (Archer).

S. Hall argues that "communities all exist based on some degree of underlying social contract—without agreement, a fundamental notion of obligation and organization, there can be no community" (p. 197). Bay suggests that a community should be understood as one in which a friendly "we-feeling" develops, and in which obligations are symmetrical and not imposed. Communities then differ by how they define their obligations. So-called minimalist communities are nonregulated groups of individuals for whom personal freedom is of the highest importance, and the only obligation to others in the community is to avoid harming them. More common is a concept of community whereby some personal freedom is given up in exchange for other goods (which may include, for example, the public health). Bellah et al. suggest that communities are what tie us to the past and the future. "They carry a context of meaning that can allow us to connect our aspirations for ourselves and those closest to us with the aspirations of a larger whole and see our own efforts as being, in part, contributions to the common good" (p. 153).

Usually an individual will belong to several communities simultaneously. For example, he or she may be a member of a family, a neighborhood, a geographic and geopolitical community, and multiple organizations and lifestyle or cultural communities. Also, a particular aggregate of individuals may form more than one type of community, and communities may overlap. A geographic neighborhood that maintains and nurtures the quality of neighboring, in which people feel that they belong, and relate to and care for their neighbors, is both a structural and an emotional community. If members of the same neighborhood share a social interest in a given issue, even something as basic as educating their children, they are also a functional community. On the other hand, there do exist aggregates of individuals in which interactions between members and a sense of common interests are lacking. Bellah et al. refer to these as "lifestyle enclaves," formed by people who share some feature of private life but are not interdependent, do not act together politically, and do not share a history (p. 335).

For the purposes of this book, several understandings of "community" are essential. First of all, developing an effective vaccine against HIV is for the benefit of communities at high risk of infection and for society at large. In order to demonstrate and establish the efficacy of a vaccine candidate, high-risk communities must be identified as indicated by a high seroincidence of infection. These are essentially structural communities, defined primarily by geography (the East Bronx, a rural village in Rwanda), culture/behavior (gay men, intravenous drug users, hemophiliacs), or organizations (sexually transmitted disease clinics, drug treatment facilities, prisons), for example. However, these "communities" may not identify themselves as such. The cooperation of large numbers of people in these communities at high risk must be obtained in order to conduct clinical research and thereby demonstrate vaccine efficacy. So members of these communities must identify themselves as part of the community, perceive themselves and their community to be at risk of infection from HIV, and be convinced that a vaccine against HIV is a good idea and something that they could and would use. This suggests that these must also be emotional communities, communities to which the individual members feel they "belong." A major challenge to researchers interested in testing HIV vaccines will be to help these communities also see themselves as functional communities that can identify a common need (to reduce the risk and incidence of HIV infection) and work together to achieve it. In this sense, they may become "communities of solution" within which a "problem can be defined, dealt with, and solved" (National Commission on Community Health Services, p. 2).

The practical realities of identifying and enlisting the cooperation of communities at high risk of HIV are formidable. Community members not only must be at high risk of infection, but also must perceive themselves to be at high risk, have a sense of belonging to the community, and accept that vaccine research is a viable yet partial solution to the problem of HIV infection. The success of vaccine trials depends on the support and cooperation of more than just potential subjects. Additionally, many of the risks and benefits of vaccine research will impact the larger community of which trial participants are a part. Before beginning vaccine trials, it is incumbent on the investigators and the research team to learn as much as they can about the target communities, including community infrastructure and characteristics, cultural groups, social and political structures, health factors, and beliefs, as well as community perceptions about research, the research team, and the sponsoring institution(s). After identifying and assessing the community, the research team should identify and establish linkages with important community contacts and leaders. This includes not only government and political leaders but also business leaders, clergy, key people in organizations and institutions, and informal leaders as well. Community-based organizations (CBOs) can be an invaluable source of information and connection with the community. As suggested earlier, investigators should hold town meetings or public forums in the community during which the purposes and processes of research can be explained and scientific, ethical, and social issues discussed. These meetings should be planned and conducted with the help of community leaders and organizations. Local media can be helpful in publicizing the meetings and in making the research visible. A community advisory board should be established for each vaccine trial, with members elected by the community to represent their needs and perspectives. The community advisory board and willing CBOs should be invited to partici-pate in writing or reviewing vaccine protocols. To the extent possible, research staff should be recruited from the community. Hiring a community outreach educator or team may be extremely useful to provide current infor-mation to the community, organize periodic meetings between the research team and community members, act as a liaison with appropriate CBOs, pro-vide in-service training to investigators and the research staff about community issues, write community-oriented educational materials, and attend appropriate community meetings. The research team and the community advisory board may work together to devise a list of the rights and responsibilities of participants and the research team. Although all of these strategies will help to establish the kind of partnership suggested above, overcoming the mistrust of researchers and the scientific establishment which is prevalent in some communities remains a major challenge to those con-ducting vaccine research.

There is another sense of community that might be tapped into: community as a normative concept, as describing a desired level of human interactions. People can be understood as communal; in fact, morality may not make sense without this understanding. People are more than coexisting autonomous individuals with rights. They relate to each other and at some level respect each other. Although some universal moral obligations may exist (such as do no harm), many moral obligations are specific and particu-lar. A person is constituted, at least in part, by his/her relations to others in the community and has a stake in sustaining the community as a good, and therefore has special obligations to members of the community (whether it be family, church, country, etc.) (Avineri and deShalit). People form ties of love and friendship, they form neighborhood associations, political parties, civic groups, churches, activist groups, etc., and they share common values and goals with others. Lacking in the current guidelines and codes of research ethics is a recognition of the value and strengths of the communi-tarian nature and values of people. Commitment to others and to the common good should be recognized, nourished, and encouraged. Guidance based only on respect for rights and avoiding harm fails to acknowledge the true richness of persons. Respect for persons should encompass more than just a respect for their ability to make autonomous choices. The role of re-search in answering socially important questions should be explicit, and communities should be empowered to help in determining what the socially important questions are.

> A prevention policy should include a place for public spirit and recognize that people sometimes do for others what they will not do for themselves. Public spirit is often heightened in times of adversity such as war. It is easy to remain self-interested when all is well, but crisis evokes a sense of public responsibility even in the complacent. AIDS is a crisis that has the potential to bring out civic virtue. (Rodwin)

HIV VACCINE

INDIVIDUAL BENEFITS AND RISKS FROM AN HIV VACCINE

As previously described, direct individual benefit from participation in vaccine research is marginal at best. With any effective vaccine, the individual is protected from the possibility of developing an infectious disease at a future time when s/he may be sufficiently exposed to the putative infectious agent. For an HIV vaccine, the benefit to the individual from a vaccine is even more provisional than with some other vaccines because in the majority of cases, HIV infection is acquired through voluntary (and avoidable) behaviors.[27] Given adequate information about how to avoid or reduce risk, many adults could prevent HIV infection in themselves without a vaccine.

The risks of an HIV vaccine for the individual may also be greater than with some other vaccines. Most vaccine research is associated with risks (1) inherent in the administration of an injection (although these are very mild and predictable); (2) of allergic or other untoward immunologic reactions to the vaccine preparation; (3) of reactions to toxic components of the vaccine (e.g., impurities, adjuvants, stabilizers); (4) of enhancement of disease (which has occurred with some viral vaccines such as respiratory syncytial virus, killed measles virus, dengue fever); and (5) of unknown side effects, which could be serious even if rare. In vaccine trials, placebo recipients, although not exposed to vaccine risks, are at risk of contracting the infectious disease—in fact, vaccine efficacy will be proven only if some do. HIV vaccine research is associated with all of those risks *plus* additional risks, including a theoretical potential for immunotoxicity or autoimmune problems from the vaccine antigens (because of the way HIV antigens bind to immune cells); a theoretical potential for integration of the viral antigens (because of the ability of HIV to integrate into cells); the potential for social discrimination and harm because of HIV antibody seroconversion, or because of participation itself; and a potential for increased risk of infection because false expectations about a (less than 100 percent effective) vaccine could result in an increase in risky behavior. "Risk of personal injury and social discrimination may make trials of candidate vaccines unjustifiable (according to Helsinki for example), unless the level of expected risk is exceedingly small" (Mariner, 1990, p. 339). Do these expected possible risks (although the frequency and magnitude is unknown; see more in chapter 4) constitute a small enough risk to justify proceeding with human research of HIV vaccine candidates? The answer to this likely will vary with the community and with the vaccine candidate.

A participant in a vaccine trial accepts immediate as well as long-term risks, both known and unknown. Most drugs have a fairly short half-life and are excreted or metabolized after a relatively short period of time (although some can do permanent damage). Vaccines work by introducing material which activates the immune system and are designed to have long-lasting effects. In some cases, as in the case of live attenuated virus, the biological material could revert and cause the infection. Activation of the immune system itself may also be harmful and is the basis of a great deal of pathology. The hoped-for long-term protection and activation of the immune system may make the effects of the vaccine "irreversible." Most codes and regulations guiding the conduct of human-subjects research require that subjects be informed that they can voluntarily withdraw from participation in the research at any time without jeopardizing their care (for example, see 45CFR.46.116(a)(8)). Participants in a vaccine trial can withdraw from the research and follow-up but may not be able to "withdraw from" or "discontinue" the effects of the vaccine, and they must be so informed. This includes, in the case of HIV, the understanding that the vaccinated individual may permanently test positive for antibody to HIV antigens induced by the vaccine, as well as the possibility that the vaccine-induced immune response may actually enhance disease. An individual vaccinated with an investigational HIV vaccine may also become ineligible for any future HIV vaccines (which, although possibly more effective, may be harmful or useless in the previously vaccinated) and/or for participation in the evaluation of future HIV vaccines (primarily because of difficulty in interpreting immune responses). Thus an HIV vaccine has a number of potential risks associated with it and would benefit only individuals who have been inadvertently exposed or have engaged in high-risk behaviors (and even then it would be a gamble with a vaccine less than 100 percent effective).

COMMUNITY BENEFITS AND RISKS OF AN HIV VACCINE

An HIV vaccine would benefit the community and the individual as a member of the community by reducing the chances of exposure to HIV, as well as by reducing the incidence of infection and the associated morbidity, mortality, and costs of HIV disease.

Potential risks to the community of testing and utilizing an HIV vaccine include the potential for an increase in risk behavior with little change in incidence because of false expectations of an only moderately effective vaccine; vaccine injury with resultant liability and a decrease in confidence about vaccines in general; difficulty in testing future, possibly more effective vaccines; the potential for wasting/diverting resources and subjecting participants to unjustified harm if a vaccine candidate is prematurely tested in humans and found to be useless or harmful (this might also result in a decrease in confidence in clinical research and/or a decrease in confidence in vaccines); the potential for loss of credibility and trust if a trial fails to provide an answer or if the community feels "deceived" or "used"; and possible exploitation of vulnerable subjects and discrimination against participants.

IMPLICATIONS OF THE COMMUNITY
MODEL FOR INDIVIDUAL INTERESTS
AND RIGHTS

Convergence of individual *interests* with community interests, as proposed, does not negate the existence of individual *rights* (for example, not to be harmed, to be informed, not to be deceived or exploited, to be treated fairly, etc.); thus it is not a utilitarian argument. As participant members who identify with the community, individuals shape and then agree with the goals of the community with respect to research, and are willing to support the conduct of research that is in the interests of the community. To do so they must be given adequate and honest information about the scientific and logistical possibilities and limitations of the proposed research. They must be treated equitably, and their deliberations, concerns, and decisions must be respected.

This model of community consultation and consent also does not imply that the "community" can dictate any and all conditions of the research. The design and conduct of the proposed research must still satisfy the principles of beneficence, respect for persons, and justice. Arbitrary decisions by some members of the community that reflect lack of respect for other members, or community negotiations about research details which are not fair to some members of the community, do not conform to an ideal of the community as a partner committed to group deliberation and decision making and mutual satisfaction of group and individual interests.

Many critics of the individualist philosophy underlying codes of research ethics have focused their concerns on the justification for, and feasibility of, informed consent. Some have suggested that the requirement for informed consent of the individual research subject cannot be universally applied because it does not always make sense based on culture and the concept of personhood (see, for example, CIOMS guidelines, 1991, 1993). In some cases it is suggested that tribal or community leaders or heads of households give consent instead of, or in addition to, the individual research subject.[28] Shifting the concept of the individual subject from a liberal view to a more communitarian view may help to reconcile problems in justifying research and in balancing risks and benefits, but it does not change the requirements for individualized informed consent, and in fact adds an *additional* requirement for community consent. Conceiving of individuals as inextricably related to and deriving identity from their community gives the individual a stake in research that is good for the community. For vaccine research especially, a system whereby consent to conduct the research was obtained from the "community" and input was obtained from the community about how to conduct it, followed by individual consent from each of the participant-subjects, should be the ideal. Such a system, in which community members would deliberate together about the ends and methods of research, would give the individual community member some responsibility in supporting the research. Such active participation in deciding the ends and the means promotes the interests of the individual and the community. However, each individual (including women!) should still maintain the right and option to decide whether or not to participate as a subject, and should be well-informed, invited to participate, and asked to consent. The influence of community decisions as potentially affecting (coercing) the decisions of individuals should be guarded against. Community input about the design and the methods of research could also serve to incorporate important cultural values or norms and thereby make the process of informed consent more appropriate to the setting.

Changes in approach to the assessment of the risks and benefits of research are not based on an increased focus on autonomy which allows the individual to define benefit and risk for him/herself and make choices accordingly (see, for example, HIV-related changes in clinical trials and the regulation of drugs, chapter 2), but rather on an increased focus on the individual as related to others and as part of a group. The group's interests are his/her interests; the group defines acceptable risks and benefits for the group and makes choices based on this. Respect for persons is understood as more than respect for their autonomy and includes respect for the wholeness of persons, their integrity, their connectedness to others, and their public-spiritedness and capacity to act in solidarity with their community. The community is given the power to evaluate the risks and benefits of research from their collective perspective and to make an informed autonomous decision about participating as a community. If the community gives consent for the research to be conducted in that community, individual members are invited to participate; they are treated fairly and with respect; and their rights are protected. Potential subjects should be well aware that the research is being done in the interests of their community. Any pretense or struggle to find a way to make the experiment potentially for the individual's direct benefit is eliminated, because it is explicit that the primary benefit is for the community. The research is understood as an attempt to evaluate a vaccine that has potential direct benefit for the community, and thus (less directly) for the individuals who make up the community.

Relevant risks and benefits to be considered in justifying research now include short- and long-term benefits and risks to individuals and the community, as perceived by the community. The community itself, as well as individual participants, can benefit or be harmed not only by whether or not research is done, and the outcomes of the research (the knowledge to be gained), but also by the way the research is conducted.

▲
_____
▼

CHAPTER FOUR

The State of
HIV Vaccine Science

In previous chapters it has been argued that having an HIV vaccine is a social good, and that human-subjects research required to find an effective one can be justified. Given this, the next question is, How should HIV vaccine research be conducted? "The obvious need for means to prevent or treat HIV infection or AIDS . . . provides strong evidence of the importance of research aimed at developing such treatment or prevention. However, it may not be possible to justify clinical testing for all investigational substances" (CIOMS, 1993, p. 39). Likewise, it is not possible to justify all methods of clinical testing.

Ethical issues pertinent to the conduct of clinical testing of HIV vaccines are complicated. Considerations of the generic issues associated with research with human subjects and the differences between vaccine research and drug research form an important background for considering the specifics of this matter. Decisions about how to conduct clinical trials for an HIV vaccine should be made in light of some of the issues and ongoing ethical controversies inherent in clinical trial methodology, as well as issues specific to HIV. The randomized controlled clinical trial (RCT) is generally recognized as the most reliable and therefore best means of proving the efficacy of vaccines, at least initially, and the ethics of the RCT has received a great deal of attention, yet some of the issues have been the subject of continued controversy. The nature of HIV, its transmission, pathogenicity, epidemiology, politics, and social reactions give rise to some ethical quandaries which are unique to HIV vaccine trials. Although some of these specific problems have been recognized and discussed in the literature, most of the discussion has occurred in isolation from some of the larger issues.

Since the intended goal of a vaccine is prevention of HIV, vaccine efficacy should ideally be evaluated within the context of a broader evaluation of methods of prevention of HIV. Because the primary beneficiary of vaccine research will be the community, communities should have the opportunity to weigh the potential risks and benefits of the research and to give their informed consent for participation. Researchers must be daring and creative in the scientific questions they ask, but careful and thoughtful about how and when they invite other human beings to be partners in the application and evaluation of the science. Decision making and review of proposed research should be performed at multiple levels.

SCIENTIFIC CHALLENGES

Despite the urgent need for an anti-HIV vaccine and the unprecedented scientific accomplishments that have occurred in the field of HIV, the development of a vaccine remains fraught with a number of challenges. HIV differs significantly from other viruses for which successful vaccines have been made. These differences have created scientific hurdles for which no parallels exist. Coupled with many only recently available scientific technologies and capabilities, this has made the scientific effort to develop an HIV vaccine extraordinary and unique. Many scientists are involved in an intense competition to design the first successful HIV vaccine, using recombinant DNA technology, hybrid viruses, synthetic peptides, and other new procedures. "Not all of the problems [involved in] developing a vaccine are because of a tricky virus, some are due to the new way science is done" (J. C. Chermann, as quoted by Challice, p. 121).

Much work is being done in the evaluation of "therapeutic" HIV vaccines, i.e., vaccines given postinfection in an effort to boost the immune system and alter the progression of disease. Clearly the science, politics, and progress in this area have an enormous impact on what happens with prophylactic vaccines. However, in many ways, issues surrounding the testing of therapeutic vaccines are materially similar to those associated with testing other forms of therapy, and so this discussion is limited to prophylactic vaccines.

HOW HIV DIFFERS FROM OTHER VACCINE-PREVENTABLE VIRAL INFECTIONS

Most diseases amenable to prevention by vaccination have a somewhat predictable sequence of steps leading to infection, disease, and protection. When a typical virus first enters the body (as free virus), it silently replicates, usually in the mucosa of the respiratory, gastrointestinal, or reproductive organs, depending on the virus. Viremia (virus in the blood) follows, with expansion and dissemination of the virus and invasion of target cells. Clinical disease occurs when enough virus has replicated and been able to in some way damage the target organ. Effective prophylactic vaccination interrupts this process at any point prior to significant viral replication in the target organ (Karzon, Bolognesi, and Koff).

Although some vaccines induce both the production of antibody and cell-mediated immune responses to a virus, the presence of persistent circulating neutralizing antibody is usually protective and is therefore accepted as a surrogate marker of protection (ibid. and others). Most viral vaccines do not completely block or prevent infection—in fact, live vaccines actually cause infection in a modified form—but they do prevent disease (Haynes; Hilleman, 1989; Karzon, Bolognesi, and Koff). Most viral vaccines currently in use protect against diseases that follow the pathogenic pattern described. Infectious diseases that do not follow this pattern (for example, those limited to mucosal sites or having a latency period) have been notoriously difficult to prevent (Dr. Daniel Hoth, Grand Rounds, National Institutes of Health, January 1993; Karzon, Bolognesi, and Koff). Most viral diseases for which there is an effective vaccine do not have a latency period, result in no significant damage to the immune system, have limited (if any) antigenic variation, and, most important, are followed by spontaneous recovery, usually with complete and long-term protection.

Although the pathogenic processes of HIV infection and disease are not completely known, the pattern is different from that described above. HIV is a member of the lentivirus family of nontransforming cytopathic retroviruses (Schooley, among others). Lentiviruses are characterized by slow, progressive infection in which virus escapes immune defenses and may cause disease after a long latency period (Katzenstein, Quinnan, and Sawyer, p. 558). Transmission of HIV occurs by virus hidden inside infected cells as well as by free virus (Hilleman, 1992). The primary point of entry into the host may be mucosal (usually vaginal or rectal) or parenteral. Replication at the mucosal site has not been described. Invasion of the target cells takes place early on, possibly before viremia occurs, and some virally infected cells are transmitted (cell-associated virus). Target cells include epithelial cells of the rectal mucosa and, most important, cells of the immune system, such as CD4 positive T cells and monocytes/macrophages. Over time, infected CD4+ T cells, normally particularly important in coordinating protective immune responses, are depleted.

HIV is composed of genomic RNA enclosed in a viral core (p24) surrounded by a viral envelope (gp160, which when split is gp120 plus gp41). The HIV envelope is hypervariable and antigenically very diverse. The envelope protein (gp120) attaches to the CD4 receptor on immune cells to gain entry into the cell. Once inside, some viral DNA integrates into the genome of the cell as a *provirus*. The cell remains infected for variable periods of time (usually years) until it is destroyed. During this variable period, many of the infected cells do not express viral antigens and are therefore undetectable by the immune system. The individual is asymptomatic for an average of ten years or more.

Although viremia occurs early in infection, it is rapidly checked by the development of antibodies and other immune responses. Low-level viremia may persist, and antigenic variants which escape immune attack emerge (Ada, Koff, and Petricciani; Karzon, Bolognesi, and Koff; Schooley). It has recently been demonstrated that despite the absence of viremia, viral burden and activity in lymph tissues is substantial (Pantaleo et al.). Antibodies are powerless against intracellular virus, and new antibodies are always needed because HIV changes constantly. Cytotoxic T lymphocytes (CD8+ T cells) in high numbers may also function to eliminate infected cells, but may become ineffective because of the ability of HIV to mutate, and because some infected cells do not express antigen. Antibodies to all parts of the virus as well as other immune responses are present, yet infection persists and the individual experiences progressive immune destruction and eventually clinical disease. The presence of neutralizing antibodies, other functional antibodies, and directed cytotoxic lymphocytes does *not* protect against the eventual development of disease. Not only are traditional immune responses *not* protective, but the virus attacks the controlling elements of the immune system and eventually destroys them, in turn setting the stage for clinical disease. Nonneutralizing HIV envelope antibodies can actually enhance HIV growth *in vitro* and might promote progression of HIV infection *in vivo* (Haynes, p. 1280). Recovery from infection has not been observed (Hilleman, 1992; Karzon, Bolognesi, and Koff).

> It is evident that with these large differences, and the absence of success stories from the past, there are no guidelines toward an AIDS vaccine. The time-proven approach of trying to mimic the immune response to natural infection makes little sense for a virus to which the natural immune response by the host fails and is ineffective. (Hilleman, 1992, p. 1054)

SCIENTIFIC APPROACHES TO MAKING A PREVENTIVE HIV VACCINE

HIV infection evokes measurable antibody and cell-mediated responses, but these do not provide protection from disease once infection has occurred (Katzenstein, Quinnan, and Sawyer, p. 561). The basic goal of prophylactic vaccine development—prevention of infection or disease—is based on the premise (and hope) that immunity as manifested by neutralizing antibodies and cell-mediated immunity, if present *before* exposure to HIV, could *prevent* virus infection, or at least *restrict disease progression* and infection transmission in those who subsequently become infected (as happens with most other viral vaccines).

Most successful viral vaccines to date have employed either live attenuated viruses (e.g., rabies, measles, mumps, rubella, poliomyelitis) or whole killed virus (e.g., influenza, Salk polio). The first, and so far only, recombinant virus vaccine is the hepatitis B vaccine, composed of recombinant hepatitis B surface antigen expressed in yeast. The hepatitis B surface antigen is a component of the hepatitis B virus known to induce the production of protective antibody. (See chapter 1 for a general discussion of vaccines.)

Specific approaches to the development of an HIV vaccine have included traditional methods but also more novel ones now possible because of advances in science and technology. Approaches have been chosen based on knowledge obtained from the study of other animal retroviruses, even though there are to date no highly effective vaccines against retroviruses that might point the way to an HIV vaccine. Approaches have also been selected because of primary considerations of safety and practicality. For some of the newer approaches there are no previous examples of success.

Traditional Approaches: Live Attenuated and Whole Killed Virus Vaccines
Attenuated live virus. Many successful viral vaccines currently in use employ live attenuated viruses. These most accurately mimic natural infection and induce the most appropriate and long-lasting immune response in diseases where recovery is associated with protection. Researchers generally believe that this strategy is not appropriate for HIV because the virus is just too dangerous.[29] Safety concerns include fear of potential reversion to pathogenic wild-type forms *in vivo*, serious side effects among persons with compromised immune systems (e.g., malnourished persons), and concerns about the presence of other HIV genes which could be integrated into host cells and have unpredictable effects (e.g., carcinogenesis). Also problematic is how to determine what is adequate attenuation (especially in the absence of an adequate animal model), as well as issues of growing enough virus under secure conditions.

Another possible live-virus approach to preparing an HIV vaccine is the use of gene-deletion techniques to produce a nonpathogenic virus. Problems with this approach include lack of understanding of pathogenic genes and the possibility that vaccine antigens could combine with endogenous pieces of retrovirus or other genes, either making the virus pathogenic or causing the growth of a tumor (Zuckerman, 1988).

Inactivated whole virus. The use of inactivated whole virus has been a successful method of making some vaccines. Inactivated whole-virus vaccines alone usually do not adequately generate an immune response, and so boosters and/or adjuvants are used to augment the response. Problems in the use of whole inactivated virus for HIV include growing enough HIV under secure conditions, purifying killed HIV (notoriously hard), completely inactivating HIV without loss of immunogenicity (and how to measure this in an animal model), and uncertainty about the dangers of cell culture systems in which HIV is grown, especially the possibility of new virus (Katzenstein, Quinnan, and Sawyer; Zuckerman, 1988). Whole inactivated HIV vaccines could also theoretically induce immunosuppression by binding with CD4 molecules on cells. Additionally, there are several previous examples of whole killed vaccines causing immune reactions which resulted in more severe clinical disease or viral enhancement after challenge with, or exposure to, virus. This occurred in goats and sheep vaccinated with whole killed retroviral preparations (Zuckerman, 1988); in kittens immunized with whole killed feline leukemia virus (FCCSET); and in humans vaccinated with whole killed respiratory syncytial virus (Beale; Chanock; Hilleman, 1989) and whole killed measles virus (Beale; Hilleman, 1989; Preblud and Katz). The use of whole inactivated virus was initially thought to be a successful approach to a simian immunodeficiency virus (SIV) vaccine in monkeys; however, the protection achieved was found, at least in part, to be the result of immune responses to the human antigens in which the SIV was grown (J. Cohen, 1992a; Schultz and Hu).

Although whole killed vaccine approaches for prophylaxis are under development, to date clinical studies with whole killed HIV have been conducted only in already infected individuals with a hope of therapeutically boosting their immune response and thereby preventing or delaying disease progression (Salk, 1987). Safety and liability concerns have limited industrial interest in whole-inactivated approaches (FCCSET).

Newer Approaches to Vaccine Development
Subunit vaccines. Most HIV vaccine candidates tested to date have been subunit vaccines using envelope antigens as the principal immunogen, either purified from virus or produced by recombinant DNA. HIV envelope is composed of two glycoproteins, gp120 and gp41, produced as a single large glycoprotein, gp160. HIV infection of cells occurs after gp120 binds to the CD4 receptor on the target cell, resulting in fusion of the membranes and entry of the virus into the cell. Theoretically, blocking the binding of gp120 to CD4 through vaccine-induced neutralizing antibody could prevent infection of the cell. Envelope proteins are also the predominant antigens expressed on the surface of infected cells in which virus is replicating. Thus cell-mediated immune responses to envelope subunit vaccines could help to clear infected cells. Nearly all infected individuals produce antibodies to gp120 and gp41; therefore they are immunogenic proteins and likely targets for an effective immune response. Experimental work with bovine leukemia virus, murine leukemia virus, and feline leukemia virus in which animals were protected by envelope vaccines provides an additional rationale for the use of envelope proteins as vaccine candidates (Katzenstein, Quinnan, and Sawyer).

The genetic information for the envelope proteins gp160, gp120, and gp41 has been cloned and introduced into yeasts, bacterial plasmids, vaccinia vectors, and vertebrate and invertebrate cells (Zuckerman, 1988). The proteins produced are recognized by the sera of HIV-infected patients. Native or recombinant envelope glycoproteins inoculated into animals cause production of measurable titers of neutralizing antibody and functional antibody and produce cytotoxic lymphocyte activity against cells expressing HIV antigens.

Using vaccines made of viral subunits has a distinct safety advantage over using whole attenuated or killed virus because infection with HIV cannot occur. However, the question remains whether subunits can sufficiently elicit an appropriate immune response (even if the appropriate immune response were known). Subunits are generally not as comprehensively immunogenic as whole virus vaccines are, even with the use of augmenting adjuvants. Further, because strains of virus seem to vary the most in the envelope, the usefulness of the immune response generated by subunit envelope vaccines may be limited. Subunit vaccines also have potential theoretical risks of their own. Viral antigens in the vaccines could themselves cause immunodeficiency or immunotoxicity (via binding to and inhibition of T4 cells), immune enhancement, or autoimmune phenomena via molecular mimicry (Hilleman, 1992; Zuckerman, 1988). In animal studies of protection, the results of subunit vaccines have been disappointing or limited (Schultz and Hu).

The majority of prophylactic HIV vaccine candidates thus far tested in Phase I clinical trials, and the only ones that have progressed to Phase II clinical trials (as of June 1994), have been subunit vaccines using envelope glycoproteins. Envelope subunit vaccine candidates are also being tested in Phase I and II trials in HIV-infected individuals with the goal of therapeutically boosting the immune response to HIV. To date, all of the subunit HIV candidates tested have induced HIV-neutralizing antibodies that last, at best, only several months after boosting (Haynes).

HIV core proteins, such as p24, stimulate anti-p24 antibody in infected individuals. Increasing core antigenemia (increasing p24) is associated with advancing disease. Theoretically, boosting antibody production to p24 could limit the rate of progression of disease. Vaccines using p24 antigen have been tested in HIV-infected individuals as a potential immunoenhancing therapy (NIAID intramural program). Two trials in which uninfected volunteers were immunized against core antigens were reported in 1992. These included HGP-30, a synthetic peptide derived from the p17 antigen and a p24 viruslike particle (p24 introduced into the yeast transposon Ty) (Fast and Walker, p. S151). Synthetic immunogens have never been used in human vaccines before, and it is unknown if they will be sufficiently immunogenic to elicit a protective response.

Hybrid virus vaccines, live recombinant virus vectors. Experiments have been done inserting HIV envelope genes into unrelated live virus vectors (e.g., vaccinia, adenovirus, herpes simplex) to create hybrid vaccines. Theoretically this approach provides the advantages of live-attenuated vaccines (i.e., closer mimicry of natural infection) with greater safety (since the genes for HIV replication are not included, there is no chance of integration and persistence of HIV in cells). Reproduction of the vector results in the production of HIV proteins.

Trials of a vaccinia-HIV envelope recombinant vaccine provided the first studies of a recombinant live vector in humans (Karzon, Bolognesi, and Koff, p. 1047) and the first studies of any HIV vaccine in humans (Zagury et al.). Use of vaccinia recombinants as the sole immunizing agent has been found to be most immunogenic in vaccinia-naive individuals (Aldovini and Young; Graham et al.). Combinations using recombinant vaccinia-HIV envelope for primary immunization followed by recombinant subunit boosters induced both neutralizing antibody and cellular immune responses at levels not previously achieved by either alone (Karzon, Bolognesi, and Koff, p. 1047). Problems with the use of vaccinia virus as a vector include the lack of laboratory markers for attenuation of vaccinia, the potential for alteration of the virulence of vaccinia, the potential for adverse reactions to vaccinia (especially in immunocompromised persons), and the possible spread of vaccinia to contacts (especially those who are immunosuppressed) (Zuckerman, 1988). The spread of vaccinia to contacts of the vaccinee could also result in the development of HIV antibodies by the contact with all of the associated implications. However, there are several advantages to this model, including low cost, ease of administration, vaccine stability, long shelf life, and the possibility of including several different antigens (Aldovini and Young; Bloom; Zuckerman, 1988).

Because vaccinia vaccine has not been widely used since the 1960s, many young adults never received it and are thus not immune to vaccinia. Safety and immunogenicity therefore are being evaluated separately in populations previously immunized with vaccinia and those not previously immunized ("vaccinia-naive"). Live recombinant adenovirus vector vaccines are also being developed. Potential theoretical advantages of this model are that the vaccine would be oral, so virus could be released in the intestine, replicate, and possibly induce mucosal immunity. It would also be easy to administer and relatively inexpensive. Recombinant adenoviruses have been used to express HIV envelope and core proteins and SIV envelope (Aldovini and Young). Phase I trials have begun.

The use of live recombinant bacterial vectors (e.g., BCG and Salmonella) to produce HIV proteins is also being explored (Aldovini and Young).

Combination vaccines. Finally, combinations of different vaccine preparations and/or antigens may play an important role in a successful vaccine strategy.

Many other experimental approaches to the development of HIV vaccine candidates are being studied and are in various stages of preclinical testing.

COMMON PROBLEMS

Scientific problems common to the development of an HIV vaccine using any approach include the lack of an understanding of the correlates of immunity, the lack of an appropriate animal model, the genetic variation of HIV isolates, and the lack of standard immunological tests for comparing responses to vaccine candidates.

What Are the Correlates of Immunity?

Deficiencies in the knowledge of pathogenesis and of what constitutes protective immunity to HIV infection or disease progression are one of the major scientific gaps impeding the development of a vaccine (Fauci et al.; Fauci; Haynes; Hilleman, 1992; Karzon, Bolognesi, and Koff; Sabin, 1992). HIV-infected persons have high titers of antibody, including antibody that is capable of neutralizing virus *in vitro*, but they are still not protected against disease progression. Hilleman's suggestion that AIDS might be a failure of the immune system to clear the infection instead of a failure to develop adequate neutralizing antibody cannot be easily dismissed (1989, p. 7).

However, the immunology of disease progression may be very different from that of protection against infection. The induction of long-lasting, broad-spectrum immunity prior to exposure to HIV is believed by many to be the best hope for effective immunization. Even though neutralizing antibodies do not prevent infected individuals from getting sick, they may have a role in preventing or altering the establishment of infection. Most of the vaccine experiments performed to date are banking on this hypothesis. Nonetheless, the capacity of antibody in human sera to neutralize HIV *in vivo* in an uninfected individual is unknown. As Sabin points out, people who have acquired infection through blood transfusion receive large amounts of antibody and still become infected; and children become infected *in utero* despite the benefit of passive maternal antibody (1992, p. 8853). In vaccine trials in animal models, there has not been a direct correlation between the presence of neutralizing antibody and protection from infection (NIAID, 1993b, p. 10; Schultz and Hu). So inducing the production of neutralizing antibody may in fact not be protective.

Little is known about the appropriate cell-mediated immune responses to aim for to protect against HIV. Additionally, the measurement of cell-mediated responses is not standard. Even if appropriate and effective cell-mediated responses could be induced and could protect against infected cells, this still might be limited to infected cells which express viral antigens on their surface and would miss intracellular virus (Sabin, 1992).

Very little is known about the role of mucosal immunity in protecting against HIV and the importance of the immune response at mucosal surfaces, yet this is potentially very important. The major mode of transmission worldwide is through sexual contact. Systemic immunity alone may be inadequate to interrupt sexual transmission of HIV. If mucosal immune mechanisms and barriers are found to be a first-line defense needed to protect against sexual transmission, what are they, and how can they be elicited or augmented? (Forrest, 1991, p. 835; Haynes). Mucosal immunity is now an active area of research (FCCSET). Even if it is determined that the induction of mucosal immunity is partially effective in blocking the contact of cells with free virus, it may not be able to prevent transmission by already virally infected cells.

It seems logical that in order to make a vaccine (which employs immunological mechanisms) to prevent against infection, one would need to understand the immunology of protection against infection or disease. It has been pointed out, however, that other vaccines have been developed without much knowledge about immune responses (Dr. Lawrence Corey, Grand Rounds, National Institutes of Health, January 1993). (For example, at the 1977 smallpox conference, 200 years after the first effective vaccine was used, researchers still did not understand the correlates of immunity.) A major difference exists, however, between previous efforts at vaccine development and the current effort to develop an HIV vaccine. In HIV the starting point is partial knowledge of the virus and its actions coupled with the scientific ability to "design" a vaccine based on this knowledge. Some of the current knowledge would be very exciting and useful if HIV behaved like an "ordinary" virus, but it does not (Hilleman, 1992). Previous vaccine work almost always started with an empirical observation about natural protection (sometimes without understanding much about the microbe; for example, even though correlates of immunity were not known, it was observed that exposure to cowpox protected people from smallpox, and this observation is what led Jenner to try his experiments), followed by attempts to copy or elicit the same type of protection using various vaccine preparations. In the absence of any observation of natural recovery from HIV in humans, there is more of a need to discover and understand the pathogenesis of HIV and the correlates of immunity in order to find an effective vaccine. Without this knowledge, the introduction of a candidate vaccine (which produces an immune response with unknown function) into humans is harder to justify and may potentially be harmful.

If specific immune responses that could protect against HIV infection or HIV-induced disease were known, development of a vaccine would be more straightforward. Candidate vaccines could be evaluated in low-risk individuals until appropriate immune responses were detected; then subsequent larger trials in high risk groups could be done with more confidence. Instead, early trials in "low-risk" individuals have evaluated traditional immune responses without knowing their significance in this disease. Inducing immune responses in individuals without knowing which are the important ones has the potential of doing more harm than good, especially for HIV because of the theoretical possibilities of immune damage and disease enhancement by vaccine antigens.

Do immune responses induced by current candidate vaccines have anything to do with prevention of infection or of disease? A vigorous research effort is underway to try to find out. This effort includes animal studies and early human studies in which immune response is being evaluated. "It is possible that identification of the critical immune responses that protect from HIV may only be determined during human vaccine efficacy studies. Thus, development of candidate vaccines in humans must be somewhat empirical" (FCCSET, p. 7).

Lack of an Adequate Animal Model

Another problem plaguing the development of an HIV vaccine is the lack of a convenient animal model for studying HIV infection and disease. Animal models have played a fundamental role in the development of vaccines against many diseases. While they may not completely represent human infection and disease, they can provide an important avenue for understanding viral replication and immune response and for evaluating the safety, immunogenicity, and efficacy of vaccine candidates before introduction into humans. This has not been true, however, for all vaccines:

> There are no meaningful animal models for measles, mumps, rubella, human adenovirus, and varicella, but clinical tests of attenuated live virus vaccines could be carried out in human beings by a "guts and judgement" approach and

without prior animal safety studies because these diseases are usually not life-threatening in their natural occurrence. Poliomyelitis, Hepatitis A and B are potentially very dangerous, but it was possible to develop *in vitro* markers and tests in susceptible animal models . . . [for] safety and protective efficacy . . . before initiating first clinical investigations. (Hilleman, 1989, p. 3)

HIV is potentially very dangerous, making a "guts and judgement" approach quite risky, yet there are as yet no suitable animal models or recognized *in vitro* markers of efficacy.

A great deal has been learned about retroviruses from studies of some animal retroviruses and lentiviruses. Particularly useful has been research with the feline immunodeficiency virus (FIV) because FIV, like HIV, targets the T lymphocyte (Karzon, Bolognesi, and Koff; Katzenstein, Quinnan, and Sawyer; IOM/NAS, 1989). Studies of primate retroviruses are particularly relevant to HIV vaccine strategies.

Simian immunodeficiency virus (SIV) is a primate retrovirus isolated from various primates, including the African green monkey. SIV infects several subspecies of monkey, causing diarrhea, wasting, CD4+ T cell depletion, opportunistic disease, and finally death. The genetic organization of SIV is similar to that of HIV-1 (and even more similar to HIV-2). To date, hundreds of macaques have been immunized with various vaccines and challenged with SIV variants (Schultz and Hu, p. 4). Most of the first SIV vaccines evaluated were whole killed virus vaccines. Some of these provided protection after challenge with SIV. In 1992, it was demonstrated that this observed protection was most likely due to immune recognition of the human antigens found in the vaccine rather than to the SIV antigens (SIV is grown in human cell lines) (ibid., p. 11). Recombinant vaccinia-SIV vaccine with subunit boosting was only sometimes successfully protective in challenge experiments on monkeys. Experiments with recombinant subunit vaccines in the SIV/macaque model have been disappointing (ibid., p. 9).

The most impressive protection against SIV challenge has been achieved by live attenuated SIV vaccines (Muthiah et al.; Schultz and Hu, p. 13). Three years after vaccination with a *nef*-deleted SIV vaccine and more than eight months after challenge with SIV, four monkeys had no signs of disease, low levels of SIV infection, and normal CD4+ cell counts, while eleven of twelve unvaccinated monkeys challenged with the same dose of virus had died (Muthiah et al.).

Intravenous challenge in animal studies is standard practice. Recently, a study demonstrated protection by inactivated SIV vaccine after intrarectal challenge; however, protection did not occur when SIV was administered intravaginally (FCCSET). Recent SIV studies have also achieved partial protection against challenge with cell-associated virus (Schultz and Hu).

The SIV model has several advantages: large breeding populations of macaques are available for medical research; they are less expensive than chimpanzees; facilities with biohazard containment conditions able to house hundreds of macaques are available in Europe and North America; and, most important, SIV infection of the macaque causes disease similar to the human disease syndrome. However, SIV is a surrogate for HIV, and it is not known whether successful SIV strategies can be translated to HIV. Additionally, there are several different SIV isolates being used in vaccine studies, and they vary quite a bit with respect to pathogenicity and other properties.

The most extensive animal HIV vaccine studies have been done in the chimpanzee, until recently the only animal in which HIV-1 can cause infection (Fischinger; Fauci; Karzon, Bolognesi, and Koff; Hilleman, 1992; IOM/NAS, 1989).[30] Chimps are readily infected by intravenous or intravaginal HIV inoculation, have a chronic infection with prolonged viremia and an immune response similar to that of humans, but *do not develop disease* or signs of T cell deficiency (Fauci; Fischinger; Katzenstein, Quinnan, and Sawyer; Karzon, Bolognesi, and Koff; Hilleman, 1992; IOM/NAS, 1989; Schultz and Hu). What happens immunologically that keeps infected chimps from developing disease is not understood, but research is being conducted to try to answer this important question (Haynes). The use of chimpanzees is also limited by their restricted availability and the high cost of their care (Fauci et al.; Haynes; Hilleman, 1989; Mariner, 1989; Schultz and Hu). Infected chimps need to be maintained in appropriate containment facilities for the rest of their lives, utilizing special and expensive long-term housing which minimizes the potential hazard of infection to animal caretakers. Because they are large, chimps require substantial housing space, and when used for research they require health care for life (forty to fifty years in captivity).[31]

To date only one HIV-1 isolate from a single challenge stock has been used to challenge chimpanzees. Other isolates either do not grow in chimps (MN) or are not yet available as challenge stocks (SF2). Efforts are being made to find stocks of other isolates that grow in chimpanzees (Schultz and Hu).

Early attempts to protect vaccinated chimps from infection with HIV failed (Fauci et al.; IOM/NAS, 1989; Mariner, 1989). Passive protection with human immunoglobulin given prophylactically also failed to prevent infection after HIV challenge; in fact, there appeared to be enhancement of infection in these animals (Hilleman, 1989, p. 5). These results were discouraging and led to great pessimism about vaccine development (IOM/NAS, 1988). Subsequent challenge studies, under ideal conditions, showed that chimpanzees can sometimes be protected from infection with laboratory strains of HIV after immunization with selected recombinant subunit vaccines (e.g., gp120 was protective, gp160 was not) (Fauci). However, this protection has occurred under very limited conditions and when the animals were challenged with virus of minimal heterogeneity. Even when a vaccine candidate is effective, the duration of protection is disappointing, and there is no protection against mucosal infection (Schultz and Hu, p. 15).

Chimps have also been protected after passive administration of monoclonal antibodies or plasma from HIV-infected persons (Karzon, Bolognesi, and Koff; Schultz and Hu). Passive protection was achieved if enough neutralizing antibody was administered immediately before or after challenge.

HIV immunoglobulin administered as soon as one hour after challenge failed to protect (Schultz and Hu, p. 8). In these studies, the successful protection achieved has been against infection by intravenous HIV. The same immunized chimpanzees challenged with intravaginal HIV become infected (Challice, p. 123). Successful experiments demonstrating protection of two vaccinated chimps challenged with infected cells to evaluate cell-associated challenge were reported in 1992 (Schultz and Hu, p. 9).

Two recent developments in the area of animal models may be potentially useful in vaccine studies. First, the HIV-1 envelope gene has been inserted into an SIV to produce a chimeric virus that can replicate in macaques (Fast and Walker; Schultz and Hu). Further evaluation of this model is needed. Secondly, the SCID *hu* mouse (a mouse without normal defense mechanisms into which elements of the human immune system are transplanted) offers an opportunity to study human immune responses to HIV and perhaps HIV vaccines, but reconstruction is imperfect (NIAID, 1993b; IOM/NAS, 1988).

The availability of a convenient and inexpensive animal model in which HIV causes disease would greatly assist in HIV vaccine development. If a candidate proved efficacious in an appropriate animal model, there would be a strong rationale for quickly developing it through large-scale human trials, even in the absence of an understanding of the specific immune responses that correlate with protection (FCCSET). The lack of a good animal model for HIV, compounded by the lack of understanding of correlates of immunity, has created disagreement as to when human efficacy studies of vaccine candidates should be initiated. Most agree that *ideally* safety, immunogenicity, and efficacy should first be demonstrated in animals. But should the lack of a suitable animal model be fatal to vaccine research? There are differences of opinion on this question. One school argues that research in humans must proceed because of the urgency of the problem, and that only by doing human trials will we obtain important information about safety, immunogenicity, and efficacy.

> With respect to HIV, lack of a convenient animal model for efficacy will mean that clinical studies of vaccines will be initiated in humans while animal studies are in progress. (Katzenstein, Quinnan, and Sawyer, p. 562)

> Some researchers feel testing in humans should await successful efficacy in chimpanzees, others that much can be learned about safety and immune response in humans before animal efficacy is attained. (Fauci et al., p. 374)

Others have argued that human testing of HIV vaccine candidates is premature, especially because of a lack of understanding of the immune correlates (Mariner, 1989; Sabin, 1992).

The argument that information about human reactions to vaccines can be obtained *only* in human studies would invalidate the general requirement for animal studies before human studies for any biological product (Mariner, 1989). If there is not a scientific reason to use evidence of safety and efficacy from animal studies, then perhaps they are not relevant. Using human subjects because they are less expensive or more convenient than chimpanzees is indefensible. Yet expense and logistics make adequate chimpanzee studies infeasible. According to one author, to really test efficacy in chimpanzees, one would have to inoculate animals at the mucosal surfaces with small amounts of virus. Given that most of them would not become infected even without a vaccine, the experiment would require approximately 100 vaccinated compared to 100 unvaccinated chimpanzees in order to reduce the infection rate in the vaccinated group to about 2 in 100 from about 8 in 100. At approximately $70,000 per chimp, this experiment could not be done (Schooley, p. 140). Whether the justification for human studies is based on the limited scientific relevance to humans of infection in chimps or on the fact that chimpanzees are too expensive or too hard to care for to be practical (or both) makes a difference. Should testing be done on humans because it is cheaper and easier, and more direct?[32] (See also Mariner, 1989, p. 87.) Perhaps the urgency of the problem coupled with the lack of a scientifically comparable animal model justifies earlier testing in humans. Karzon, Bolognesi, and Koff suggest that the problem is less that available animal models are not suitable than that the biological questions and the behavior of the virus are so complicated (p. 1044). Haynes also notes that the two problems are related and states that because of the lack of an animal model of human AIDS, and the lack of a cohort of persons naturally resistant to HIV, the immune correlates are not known. Without knowing what constitutes protection, testing in humans is more dangerous. Fundamentally, we need to know what protection is, and one way to determine that would be in an animal model that mimics human infection. Without either, how can vaccine candidates justifiably be tested in humans? "In my judgement the available data provide no basis for testing any experimental vaccine in human beings or for expecting that any HIV vaccine could be effective in human beings" (Sabin, 1992, p. 8854).

Because of the urgency of the public health need and public attention and political pressure, human Phase I trials of HIV candidate vaccines began before efficacy was demonstrated in chimpanzees or any other animal model. Phase II trials of envelope subunit vaccines have begun despite limited protection under controlled conditions provided by these vaccines in chimps and the lack of protection afforded in the SIV/macaque model. Controversy still exists as to when Phase III efficacy trials in human subjects should begin (see chapter 5).

Virus Variation
Another challenge to vaccine development is the presence of distinct HIV strains in different geographical areas. At least five to seven major virus subgroups have been defined worldwide (Karzon, Bolognesi, and Koff). A truly utilitarian vaccine should be able to stimulate broadly cross-reactive immunity against a large number of variant strains of HIV. Short of this, vaccine candidates should be developed which protect against the predominant strains in the particular areas where testing is to occur (and where vaccine will be utilized).

In addition to geographic variation, different HIV isolates have been found in different individuals within the same geographic region, and even in a single infected individual (FCCSET). Most of the variation among individual strains of virus is in the envelope proteins. This is especially a problem if the vaccine candidate uses envelope glycoproteins as the immunizing agent, as many do. Internal structural core proteins are less able to accommodate change (ibid.).

Studies are being conducted to attempt to define the genetic variation that exists throughout the world. This is important to understanding and controlling HIV, because different strains often have different pathogenic potential, affinity for cell types, and possibly even routes of entry into cells. However, little information is yet available to understand (1) the relationship of HIV genotype to the ability to cause disease; (2) the physiologic differences in terms of HIV transmissibility, rates of clinical evolution of disease, or response to therapy; and (3) the natural history of end-stage disease (ibid.). HIV isolates as much as 40 percent different in envelope genes have been identified (ibid.).[33] The World Health Organization Global Programme on AIDS (WHO/GPA) has created a network for HIV isolation and characterization. Sample strains from recent seroconverters at potential AIDS vaccine field trial sites are systematically isolated and characterized at GPA-coordinated laboratories, and the data are linked with data banks in developed countries.

Whereas in other regions several subtypes might exist, one subclass of virus is prevalent in the U.S. population. However, even within this subtype, differences in envelope gene sequence exist (as much as 15 percent). Further research is needed to attempt to classify virus types based on functional criteria. Initial vaccine candidates were based on sequences (LAI or IIIB) found to infect only a small proportion of individuals in the U.S. and Europe; more recent products are based on isolates representative of that predominantly infecting U.S. and European populations (i.e., MN and SF2 strains) (J. Cohen, 1993). Products based on isolates from other parts of the world are being developed, as are vaccine "cocktails" designed to protect against several different strains.

A vaccine which is efficacious against only one subtype of virus could slow the epidemic but not eradicate it in any given country. If a vaccine protected against some or most but not all strains, evaluation of efficacy could also be complicated if the vaccinee became infected with another strain, one which the vaccine was not designed to protect against. Genomic variability among HIV isolates (geographic and personal) may also enable the virus to escape the immune system and to infect different cells or adapt to a different environment, making the development of an effective vaccine very challenging (FCCSET).

In addition to variation in isolates, field isolates of HIV behave differently in immunological assays and in other characteristics than laboratory strains, also complicating the evaluation of candidate vaccines (Karzon, Bolognesi, and Koff, p. 1047). What is needed is a vaccine capable of inhibiting a spectrum of field isolates, not just laboratory strains of virus.

Lack of Standard Immunological Assays
Not all Phase I trials of HIV vaccines have been conducted using standard, re-
producible assays for functional immune responses (Karzon, Bolognesi, and
Koff). This has made the comparison of candidate vaccines difficult, if not
meaningless. Measurement of immune response is one of the first indicators
that a vaccine might be effective. By regulation, a vaccine must be shown to
be immunogenic in order to move forward in clinical trials. The possibility
also exists that altering the immune response to HIV may ultimately have a
deleterious effect on the course of infection (Fauci). So standard measurement
and documentation of immune responses elicited and modified by vaccine
candidates is critical in the evaluation of their safety and efficacy. Decisions
about a vaccine candidate's usefulness are made primarily on the basis of its
ability to elicit an appropriate and lasting immune response while not causing
intolerable side effects. If the immune response elicited cannot be interpreted
or reproduced by others doing similar work, there will be no basis for comparison. Likewise, if the theoretical immune damage or possibility of viral
enhancement cannot be measured in a standard way, it will be impossible to
say that these harmful effects have not occurred and that the vaccine is safe.
These possibilities strongly argue for carefully controlled clinical trials that
include monitoring of immune responses in a standardized way with subsequent comparison of the findings, as well as for comparative trials in which
several vaccine candidates are tested simultaneously.

The AIDS Vaccine Evaluation Group (AVEG, an NIAID extramural infrastructure for evaluating HIV vaccines in Phase I and II trials) performs
some routine immunological evaluation, and also employs a Central Immunology Lab for some standard immune assays (NIAID, 1992, p. 5). The
NIAID states that "standardized methodology for the measurement of
immune responses, including cell-mediated cytotoxic lymphocytes, and mucosal immune responses will continue to be developed and implemented to
ensure that complete immunological evaluation is accomplished" (ibid., p. 6).

STATE OF HIV VACCINE
CLINICAL TESTING

As described in chapter 1, vaccines are usu-
ally tested in human subjects in sequential phases. Normally all phases of
clinical research are preceded by successful evaluations of safety, immunogenicity, and efficacy in laboratory studies and animal studies. For HIV
vaccine candidates, laboratory studies, animal studies, and Phase I human
studies are being conducted in parallel.

The First HIV Vaccine Studies in Humans
In November 1986, a French scientist, Dr. Daniel Zagury, tested the first
HIV vaccine candidate (a vaccinia recombinant expressing gp160) in

humans. Dr Zagury first injected himself and then eighteen seronegative "volunteers" with his experimental vaccine. Although the fact was unreported by Dr. Zagury in his scientific publications, the volunteers were actually healthy seronegative Zairian children (ten children between two and nine years of age, and eight between ten and eighteen years) (Office for Protection from Research Risks [OPRR], Final Report: Investigation of Noncompliance with DHHS Regulations for the Protection of Human Research Subjects Involving the National Institutes of Health Intramural Research Program, March 26, 1993). According to Dr. Zagury, the children were permitted to participate on a "humanitarian" basis at the urgent request of their mothers, all of whom had AIDS themselves. In published reports of the experiments, Dr. Zagury states: "All our work in Zaire has the full support of the Zairian Ethics Committee" (Zagury et al., p. 250). In none of the publications was it mentioned that the participants were children or how they were recruited. An anonymous source close to the involved investigators said that a major reason the trial was conducted in Zaire was that "it was easier to get official permission [in Zaire] than in France" (*New York Times*, February 8, 1987, p. A1).

This experiment, when brought to the attention of the Office for Protection from Research Risks of the NIH, resulted in a series of investigations by the NIH and the French government and NIH sanctions against those involved; it also led to a reorganization of the review, approval, and oversight of intramural research (including collaborative research) conducted by NIH investigators. These experiments received much publicity and generated great controversy because of alleged deviation from ethical standards and procedures of the NIH/DHHS, accompanied by competing claims that all the ethical standards in place in France and Zaire were complied with (OPRR Report, March 1993).

Regardless of whether the standards and regulations were adhered to or deviated from, the use of children in these vaccine experiments was not justified. "This example indicates how easily ethical considerations can be swept aside under the rubric of 'humanitarianism' or 'compassion.' The children [involved] had escaped perinatal transmission; they were not at risk through casual contact with their mothers. There could be no possible benefit to them and there was potentially serious harm" (C. Levine, 1991b). These experiments represent an unfortunate beginning for the HIV vaccine effort, perhaps especially in the conduct of collaborative international research. Dr. Zagury and colleagues were severely criticized by the OPRR for these experiments, but were exonerated by French authorities. No comment was made by the Zairian government.

Phase I Studies
Phase I vaccine trials aim to evaluate safety and immunogenicity of various doses of vaccine in a small number (usually less than 100) of healthy, low-risk volunteers. Traditionally, control groups are not included in Phase I studies

because the outcomes of interest are not usually seen without vaccination (Smith, Hayes, and Mulder, p. 106). Phase I trials of HIV vaccines undertaken to date have studied the safety of various candidates and attempted to characterize the type, magnitude, and duration of immune response in low-risk individuals. Low-risk individuals are chosen to avoid including those already infected or those likely to become infected during the trial. This is done to ensure sensitivity to vaccine effects and to minimize immunologic variability (Sawyer, Katzenstein, and Quinnan). Also, we "don't want a potentially useful vaccine to be discarded because of HIV manifestations that are really from infection" (Schooley, p. 142). In Phase I HIV vaccine trials, risk has been determined by careful screening and questioning.

As of March 1993, more than twenty vaccine candidates had been or were being evaluated in a number of Phase I studies in seronegative volunteers in the U.S., Europe, and Africa (Fast and Walker; NIAID, 1992). Most of these have been gp120 or gp160 envelope subunit vaccines, but vaccinia-envelope recombinants, a core peptide vaccine (HGP30), and a particle vaccine (Ty-gag) have also entered Phase I trials. The majority of trial participants have been white males (NIAID, 1992). Many volunteers have been identified as homosexual but have been recruited as "low-risk" based on self-reported behaviors or promises made to refrain from high-risk behaviors for a period of time surrounding the vaccine trial[34] (Schooley, p. 142). Politically, it was believed it would be difficult to recruit exclusively truly low-risk individuals because individuals at risk expressed a strong desire to be part of any vaccine effort, and also it was unclear whether an adequate number of others would be forthcoming.

Some of the Phase I HIV vaccine trials have been placebo-controlled and randomized in order to better evaluate the theoretical adverse immunological effects (because of the potential for immunotoxicity and variable measures of immune function) (Sawyer, Katzenstein, and Quinnan, p. 40). Others were more traditional dose-escalating Phase I studies.

So far, all vaccine candidates evaluated in Phase I trials in seronegative individuals have appeared to be safe and well tolerated (Fast and Walker; NIAID, 1992). Evidence of long-term side effects and safety in children, pregnant women, or persons with low CD4+ T cell counts is not yet available. Observed side effects include local pain and tenderness, low-grade fever, and minor systemic symptoms, some of which also occurred in the placebo recipients. Declines in CD4+ T cell count, a theoretical concern because of potential binding of vaccine antigens to CD4+ cells, have not been observed over a follow-up period of up to twenty months or more. Other major toxicities (e.g., renal, hepatic, or neurologic) were also not observed. The possibility that antibody generated by the vaccine may actually stimulate more viral reproduction is difficult to evaluate, and may be known only when a certain number of vaccinated individuals are exposed to natural virus. Immune responses noted in the majority of vaccinated subjects include binding antibodies; low titers of neutralizing antibody to homologous virus (although comparable to antibody titers seen in gp120-vaccinated chimps protected from intravenous homologous viral challenge); low to nonexistent titers of neutralizing antibody to heterologous virus; short duration of antibody response (i.e., weeks to months, not years); and cell-mediated CD8 cytotoxic response only to combination vaccine (NIAID, 1993). Not very encouraging immunologic data!

In summary, HIV vaccine candidates so far appear to be safe, but are they useful? Data show that these vaccine candidates do not even consistently produce immune responses (and even less of sustained duration) which are believed to be useful, such as neutralizing antibody. Nonetheless, based primarily on their ability to elicit neutralizing antibodies, Phase II trials of two subunit candidates began in early 1993.

Phase II Studies
Phase II trials aim to obtain further information on safety, especially milder and less frequent reactions to vaccine; to characterize the immune response in more detail, including the duration of response; and to work out an effective and convenient dosage regimen in a larger and broader group of subjects. It is generally recommended that Phase II trials study primarily those at low risk of infection (because infection could distort the safety and immune response data) (Smith, Hayes, and Mulder), but include some subjects at high risk of infection (to be able to identify safety issues that may be unique to populations at high risk) (Porter, Glass, and Koff).

The first Phase II clinical trials of experimental vaccines to prevent HIV in seronegative persons began in January 1993 in five U.S. cities through the network of the AIDS Vaccine Evaluation Units sponsored by the NIAID. These trials are evaluating two genetically engineered gp120 subunit vaccines, derived from the two most common HIV strains in the U.S. (HIV-1 M and HIV-1-SF2), made in mammalian cells, and to which adjuvants have been added (NIAID press release, "First HIV Vaccines Move into Phase II Testing in Uninfected Volunteers," December 1, 1992). The goal is to recruit 330 seronegative men and women between the ages of 16 and 60 from diverse populations. To this end, and to encourage "minorities and people representing several different populations hardest hit by the epidemic," the eligibility criteria are less restrictive than those of Phase I trials (ibid.). One newspaper article noted that the "government is recruiting IV drug users because they are among the most likely to become infected" (Huntly, p. A1).[35] The trial design is randomized, placebo-controlled, and blind. All participants are to receive a primary vaccination and two boosters. The placebo group will be injected with adjuvant. All participants will be counseled to avoid risk behaviors. Volunteers (at Johns Hopkins University) are being paid $20 per visit to cover expenses (Huntly).

Recent studies have demonstrated consistent induction of HIV-neutralizing and syncytium-inhibiting antibodies by a recombinant envelope subunit protein vaccine (Genentech's IIIB-rgp120/HIV-1) at higher titers than previously achieved (Schwartz et al.). These findings have encouraged discussions of moving forward to Phase III efficacy trials, especially since this same gp120 product is currently being evaluated in Phase II studies. "The design of HIV vaccine Phase III efficacy trials has posed major social, ethical and logistic problems" (Haynes, p. 1283).

CHAPTER FIVE

▲
_____
▼

Planning Phase III HIV Vaccine Efficacy Trials

CONSIDERATIONS FOR EFFICACY TRIALS

Phase III trials aim to evaluate the efficacy of a vaccine in preventing infection or disease. These trials are usually randomized, controlled, blind, longer in duration than earlier-phase trials, and include a much larger sample population. Because individuals differ in their risk of disease as a result of many factors, randomization distributes these factors similarly between the group receiving the vaccine candidate and a control group. Blinding the study is useful because knowledge of vaccine status may influence an individual's risk behavior and destroy the comparability of groups (Katzenstein, Quinnan, and Sawyer; Smith, Hayes, and Mulder). Phase III efficacy trials for HIV vaccine(s) are projected to take many years to complete and to include many thousands of subjects from all of the target groups worldwide. Although there is strong pressure from many corners to test an HIV vaccine for efficacy, to date there seems to be scientific consensus that no current candidate is ready for evaluation in large-scale efficacy trials in the U.S. (AIDS Research Advisory Council, June 1994; NIAID Ad Hoc Panel, September 1992; Haynes; Hilleman, 1992; Fast and Walker; Sabin, 1992; Vermund).

A consideration of the ethical conduct of Phase III trials for vaccine efficacy should address questions of when such studies should begin, who should be included as subjects, how the studies should be done (i.e., design and logistics), and the processes which should be utilized in negotiating and reviewing scientific and ethical aspects of such studies.

Although it is essential, proving efficacy for a vaccine against HIV is inevitably going to be extremely difficult. The variable incidence of infection, the groups in which the highest incidence is found, the erratic behavior of the virus, the obligation to educate or counsel participants about risk-reductive behaviors, the influence of behavior changes, the long incubation period until development of clinical disease, the cost and length required for a traditional field trial for efficacy, and multiple political influences all complicate the problem. Proving the efficacy of any vaccine is complicated, but a high incidence of infection (such as cholera in Bangladesh), a predictable course (such as exposure to influenza in the late winter with clinical disease quickly following), knowledge about protective immune responses (such as HBsAg protecting against infection with hepatitis B), more uniform susceptibility (such as to measles or pertussis), and a lack of known methods of altering the "natural" state (i.e., no knowledge about how to reduce risk, for example, with behavior changes, sanitation, or another vaccine) all facilitate the determination of vaccine efficacy. Recognition of the realities of global incidence, variable political will, scientific competition, and difficulties in proving efficacy may set the stage for suggesting radical alternatives in HIV to the normal processes of proving efficacy. "Our backs are getting to the wall in a dramatic and dangerous situation. We will need to be ready to accept some radical approaches" (Ron Derosiers, as quoted by J. Cohen, 1992a, p. 1881). Among the suggestions are to recruit volunteers willing to be artificially challenged with live virus; to test death-row inmates; to recruit a susceptible African village to be vaccinated (without telling them it is "experimental"); not to offer any counseling or education about risk reduction; to test multiple candidates on a large scale now, without further data, in order to obtain answers; or to give up the entire endeavor as too costly and complicated and therefore not practical or worth doing. Although there can be a place for radical approaches to difficult problems, none of these suggestions is an acceptable solution because each of them shows profound disrespect for the communities and individuals who would be involved in the research.

WHEN SHOULD
EFFICACY TRIALS BEGIN?

There is disagreement in the scientific community as to when efficacy trials of preventive HIV vaccine candidates should begin (see also the discussion with respect to lack of an adequate animal model in chapter 4). It is generally agreed that "Phase III trials are only conducted if a candidate vaccine has successfully passed through Phase I and II trials" (Smith, Hayes, and Mulder, p. 106). But what does "successfully" mean in this context? What must we have learned from Phase I and II studies in order to justify proceeding? Certainly, safety is of primary importance. Although the available evidence is incomplete, it appears that most of the vaccine candidates tested in Phase I trials are safe. Secondly, some evidence of immunogenicity and ability to induce the intended effect is desirable (usually obtained from Phase I and II trials). At present, this is the crux of the disagreement. Most vaccine candidates evaluated thus far are immunogenic, although some are more so than others. However, the relationship of the induced immune response to protection against disease or infection is unclear. The value of animal studies in clarifying this relationship is limited. So, although evidence of protective efficacy from animals or early human studies is usually required before large-scale efficacy trials are conducted, this evidence may not be attainable in HIV infection.

More extensive Phase II evaluation of selected vaccine candidates will contribute to evidence of effect (or lack thereof). The careful conduct of selected Phase II studies should proceed without delay. The resultant data will also facilitate choosing among the available candidates, so that only the appropriate or best will proceed to large-scale trials. This point is extremely important given the limited resources to spend on this problem. Concurrent Phase I and II (and maybe III) trials of vaccine candidates as therapeutic immunotherapy will provide additional valuable data about safety and immunogenicity. Political pressure to find a vaccine could prompt testing for efficacy prematurely, testing too many, or the wrong, candidates. "In an atmosphere of pressure, there can be misadventure" (Gostin, 1987, p. 9). Such a misstep could have major negative consequences. An important and recent example of the power of political pressure occurred with gp160 therapeutic trials. As one person said, it was the first time that a clinical trial was designed by a congressional appropriations committee instead of scientists (Jesse Dobson, NIAID Ad Hoc Panel, September 1992).[36]

There have been numerous scientific meetings to consider criteria for the entry of vaccine candidates into efficacy trials. Although some have promised that such trials will begin soon[37] and that there will be a vaccine by the turn of the century, this is a hope, not a fact. (Dr. Margaret Heckler, former secretary of Health and Human Services, publicly promised on April 23, 1984, that we would have an HIV vaccine by the mid-1980s!). Reports from the 9th International Conference on AIDS (June 1993) again reiterated the hope that "vaccine trials may begin as early as 1994" (*AIDS Weekly*, June 14, 1993, p. 15). However, this hope was derived from an address by Dr. Dani Bolognesi in which he said: "It is prudent to establish an infrastructure . . . specifically to be prepared to implement such trials in 1994 or early 1995 *should one or more products be ready for testing*" (as quoted by the *AIDS Weekly*, June 14, 1993; my emphasis).

In July 1991, at the request of the NIAID, an ad hoc HIV Vaccine Advisory Panel met to address issues related to NIAID's role in HIV vaccine development. After extensive deliberation, the panel developed "Optimal Guidelines"[38] for entrance of a candidate vaccine into efficacy trials. These guidelines define the "ideal" prophylactic HIV vaccine. Recognizing, however, that the urgency of the HIV pandemic might necessitate entering candidates into trials before optimal guidelines could be met, the panel also established less stringent "Core Guidelines."[39] To date, no vaccine candidate has met even the core guidelines. In September 1992, an HIV Vaccine Development Workshop, also sponsored by NIAID, met to reevaluate the optimal guidelines, and to advise on scientific direction and policies concerning the development and testing of HIV vaccines. This panel reaffirmed the need for clear, concise, and well-disseminated guidelines supported by the scientific community. They recommended that these guidelines be disseminated for the study of vaccines rather than as criteria for entry into efficacy trials, and that decisions regarding the selection of individual candidate vaccines for entry into efficacy trials be made on a case-by-case basis, relative to an evolving state of the art. This panel concluded that there were insufficient data to support selection of a vaccine candidate for efficacy trials at that time and recommended the formation of a Vaccine Working Group to assist in the coordination and prioritization of vaccine research efforts.

The Vaccine Working Group, consisting of extramural investigators, constituency members, and government scientists, met for the first time in December 1992 and again in March and July 1993. The group is working with NIAID's Division of AIDS to assess the status of HIV vaccine research, identify critical questions to be addressed (scientific and otherwise), and identify priorities and mechanisms to answer those questions (NIAID, Charge to HIV Vaccine Working Group, December 1992). The Working Group will accomplish specific tasks through seven small focus groups, one of which is identified as "Efficacy Trials."[40]

A January 1993 report of the Federal Coordinating Committee on Science, Engineering, and Technology's Working Group on HIV Vaccine Development suggested two broad categories of selection criteria for candidate vaccines advancing to field trials: *in vitro* results (e.g., sustained antibody or other detectable and relevant immune response) from Phase I human studies, and *in vivo* demonstrated efficacy in model systems (e.g., HIV in chimps or SIV in macaques) (p. 65).

Many believe that despite the scientific hurdles yet to be overcome, proceeding soon with efficacy trials is justified because of the urgency of the situation:

> The time has now arrived to consider seriously the early initiation of Phase III efficacy trials in selected populations with the most promising of current candidate vaccines. There are powerful reasons for such a decision: 1) a vaccine is potentially the most efficient and cost-effective way to prevent infection and possibly to slow down progression of disease in those already infected; 2) this action would be seen publicly as a demonstration that there is a major international effort to develop HIV vaccines and the most promising ones are now ready for testing for efficacy in humans; 3) (and not least,) we are bound to learn something which will be useful in further vaccines, such as the need for broad antigen specificity, for strong, local mucosal immunity. (Ada, Koff, and Petricciani, p. 1318)

This argument as a justification for proceeding immediately is flawed. Reasons 1 and 2 are legitimate only if the outcome is good. Vaccines are certainly efficient and cost-effective if they work, but this is not a reason to test a candidate for efficacy in humans unless there is some reason (such as scientific evidence) to believe it is likely to work. This is similar in some ways to the argument from hope (see Macklin and Friedland) that HIV-infected people should have early access to experimental drugs because they need treatment (and hope) for their life-threatening illness (true, but they receive "treatment" only if the drug works). Reason 2 also supports going ahead only if the outcome is good, because testing vaccine candidates could also have devastating negative consequences. If testing a vaccine in a large number of healthy people does nothing or actually causes harm, there could be a loss of public confidence in medical research, in HIV-related research, and in vaccine programs, as well as a wasting of finite human and economic resources. Moreover, many of the groups in which vaccine trials might be undertaken already have a strong sense of distrust toward the research establishment (e.g., African-Americans because of the legacy of Tuskegee). The third reason is the only logical reason to move forward now. However, if the goal is to learn something about human immune responses, the trials should not be called vaccine efficacy trials, but should honestly be presented as efforts to learn about protective immune responses in HIV, much of which can probably be learned in smaller Phase II trials.[41] Describing the research as a way to learn more about immune responses and protection is especially important because of the significance of the word *vaccine,* which may be understood as meaning "protection" and "safety" by many people.

Petricciani also argues for moving forward now:

> Proceeding cautiously with clinical efficacy trials should not be considered adventurism, but rather a pragmatic approach to gain the most meaningful type of information as soon as possible. It is the way to progress in the best tradition of past vaccine efforts such as those against smallpox, rabies, and polio. The world is a healthier place today because individuals took the initiative to move ahead and learn from clinical studies. . . . The time for elegant studies and perfection is past, sights must be set on practical targets—not idealized goals. (Petricciani, Koff, and Ada, p. 1529)

However, the historical success of smallpox, rabies, and polio vaccines also does not justify early or premature clinical studies of efficacy. Judgment of those previous efforts is colored by outcome; all were ultimately successful, and therefore the efforts and courage of the involved scientists have been judged favorably. Nevertheless, controversy exists over the ethics of the clinical studies that were performed in the evaluation of all three examples cited. Petricciani argues for a pragmatic approach and "practical targets," both of which might affirm the need for testing of something likely to have the desired effect. If, again, the goal is really to learn more about immune responses (which is a practical target), research should be billed as such.

The sense of urgency has also been expressed in more moving ways. For example, Dr. Robert Levine, speaking at an Institute of Medicine meeting in December 1992, quoted an unnamed minister of health from a developing country with a high incidence of HIV as saying: "If you don't get on with this [testing preventive vaccines] soon, there won't be many people left in the country to protect."

Nonetheless, most, even those who favor testing human subjects in Phase I and II trials, are reluctant to proceed to Phase III studies without some evidence of a vaccine candidate's effectiveness in animals (FCCSET) or in early clinical studies (see, among others, ibid.; Hilleman, 1992; Sabin, 1992). The question remains, given the urgency of the public health problem (at least in some communities or regions), what kind and how much evidence is needed? In most cases, this determination will be made by national regulatory agencies;[42] however, the power of political pressure cannot be denied. "It need hardly be emphasized that any candidate vaccine must be subjected to meticulous evaluation, and premature unsubstantiated claims may result in loss of confidence by the public and may have a serious impact on other immunization programs" (Zuckerman, 1988, p. 383).

The Declaration of Helsinki states: "Biomedical research involving human subjects must conform to generally accepted scientific principles and should be based on adequately performed laboratory and animal experiments and on a thorough knowledge of the scientific literature." In keeping with this guideline, a decision about when to proceed to a large-scale efficacy trial with any particular vaccine candidate should be based on science. Given the limitations of animal models and laboratory tests in obtaining evidence of an HIV vaccine candidate's effectiveness, decisions about what experiments are adequate might differ from those made with regard to other diseases or infections. However, scientific principles and the usual path of laboratory, animal, and then human testing argue strongly for some evidence of desired effect (the ability to induce a *sustainable* and *relevant* immune response) before proceeding to test large numbers of healthy people. Additionally, the limited number of trial sites and the enormous costs and complexity of efficacy trials argue for careful selection of promising vaccine candidates. At this juncture, the best approach (and the one most considerate of the indispensable human and material resources) appears to be to continue aggressive efforts at the preclinical and Phase I level; move to Phase II trials a few more vaccine candidates, carefully selected based on ability to be immunogenic; conduct research specifically to try to better understand protective immune responses;[43] conduct research to better evaluate other means of prevention (such as virucides, treatment of STDs, condom use, non-reusable needles, etc.); continue infrastructure building in preparation for large-scale efficacy studies; conduct preliminary research (i.e., seroprevalence studies, behavioral studies, feasibility studies); and wait until there is some evidence of a vaccine candidate's ability to protect (and against relevant strains) before doing a large-scale "efficacy" trial.

When evidence is available, an honest comparative evaluation of all of the preclinical, animal, and early clinical work should be undertaken by a group of qualified and uninvested[44] scientists and be presented to the appropriate national authorities and the target communities along with the scientific reasons to proceed and the uncertainties. The communities will then decide whether they are willing to participate in research of this type. Some pressed by more urgent needs may opt to go ahead earlier with less evidence of effect, while others may move more cautiously, and that is fine. A community to be studied should have an opportunity for adequate review and understanding of available data, negotiating power about adequate means of protecting the rights and welfare of individual participants within the community, and the opportunity to give its collective consent. This requires that the real hopes, expectations, uncertainties, and fears of doing the research with this candidate at this time for this purpose are presented in an honest and understandable manner by the investigators. If community education and negotiation occur after governmental or regional approval is obtained but before IRB approval is sought, the community can influence the design and procedures of a particular study before it is approved.

Besides testing individual vaccine candidates for efficacy, researchers will need to conduct trials that compare the efficacy of different candidates, that evaluate the efficacy of vaccine "cocktails," and that study differences in efficacy between risk groups. Efficacy may differ between homosexual men, intravenous drug users, female prostitutes, heterosexual partners of infected men or women, or children born to infected women. It may also differ, and therefore should also be evaluated, with respect to mechanisms of transmission, geographic location, and strain variability, as well as the presence of STDs or other comorbidity (Sawyer, Katzenstein, and Quinnan, p. 40). An efficacy trial conducted in one community will need to be compared with similar trials conducted in other communities.

The scientific hurdles encountered and the scientific effort involved in developing an HIV vaccine are unprecedented. Although an enormous amount has been learned, there are still many important unanswered scientific questions which make the development of an effective vaccine possibly years away. Although there is more scientific optimism than there was two years ago, there is still a long way to go. The situation seems best summed up in the words of Dr. Maurice Hilleman:

> On the one hand, it seems a reasonable judgement that no thoughtful and responsible person could consider discontinuing the present and future work on vaccine, since the future is unpredictable. On the other hand, it is also a reasonable judgement that no thoughtful and informed person can believe or be certain that the present work on vaccine, and that planned for the future, is sufficient and has a reasonable or certain chance to provide the successful AIDS vaccine. (1992a, p. 1057)

Besides scientific criteria for starting efficacy trials, other considerations such as cost, location, endpoint measurement, subject selection, need for facilities, infrastructure, health care, protection of subjects, liability and compensation, and subsequent utilization must be dealt with. A team of researchers at the 9th International Conference on AIDS strongly urged other scientists, government leaders, and drug companies to address important social and ethical issues *before* initiating large-scale efficacy trials (Lurie et al.). Although their focus of concern was trials in developing countries, many of the same issues must be dealt with for domestic trials. Addressing these concerns should be an ongoing process while we await the availability of an appropriate vaccine candidate.

The NIAID is in the process of developing an infrastructure for the conduct of Phase III efficacy trials of HIV vaccine candidates so that when a candidate is ready for testing, the groundwork will be in place. This effort includes evaluating seroincidence, risk factors, and risk-reduction efforts in domestic cohorts of high-risk individuals; supporting similar efforts internationally through grants and the creation of PAVES (Preparation for AIDS Vaccine Evaluation Sites); and establishing (goal 1993–1994) an HIV Vaccine Efficacy Trials Network to conduct prevention research and provide the capability of doing efficacy trials (NIAID, 1993b). Several advisory groups provide broad oversight of the NIAID vaccine effort, including the Vaccine Subcommittee of the AIDS Research Advisory Committee, the AIDS Program Advisory Committee, and the National Allergy and Infectious Diseases Advisory Council. An HIV Vaccine Working Group was established in December 1992 to assist in the coordination and prioritization of HIV vaccine efforts of the NIAID. The National Cancer Institute (NCI) is also involved in basic vaccine research and primate studies. The Department of Defense (DOD) supports studies of viral variation, the clinical testing of therapeutic vaccines in infected individuals (first Phase II therapeutic vaccine trials are being conducted by Walter Reed Army investigators), and prevention in uninfected individuals. The Public Health Service and the DOD coordinate efforts with each other and with the pharmaceutical industry. Social and ethical issues are just beginning to be explored.

The WHO/GPA is also providing funding and direction for infrastructure development, staff training, and the purchase of equipment, with the goal of providing an environment for collaborative vaccine efficacy trials, both national and international. The WHO/GPA is assisting national authorities and scientists from developing countries to strengthen the infrastructure that will be required for the conduct of trials with high scientific and ethical standards. WHO-sponsored plans for HIV vaccine development have been prepared in Brazil, Rwanda, Thailand, and Uganda.[45] Each of the four countries recommended by the GPA Steering Committee is developing a national plan specifying its unique needs and recommendations (WHO/GPA). The WHO/GPA Steering Committee on Vaccine Development has also developed criteria for admission of candidate vaccines to clinical trials, especially where they are to be tested in developing countries (Esparza et al., 1991).

> WHO/GPA has taken the lead in promoting an environment which is conducive to global coordination and, where possible, collaboration in the research, development, and distribution of HIV drugs and vaccines. . . . Specific examples [include] the Steering Committee on Vaccine Development, the Network for HIV Isolation and Characterization, and the WHO-IFMPA [International Federation of Pharmaceutical Manufacturers Association] Joint Working Group. Each of these groups brings together international experts representing multiple technical areas relevant to providing guidance on conducting international HIV vaccine trials. (FCCSET, p. 62)

It is critical that Phase III trials provide reliable results upon which to base practice and improve public health. Therefore trials must be carefully designed with adequate samples and a clear sense of what "efficacy" means. Decisions must be made as to the goal of vaccination and what endpoints will be sought and measured. Is the goal of HIV vaccination for uninfected individuals complete protection from infection, or prevention of clinical disease?[46] Many believe that because of the complex behavior of the virus, its ability to integrate into host cells, and its lifelong persistence, the ideal HIV vaccine should provide complete "sterilizing" protection. But no other viral vaccine completely protects against infection (FCCSET; Haynes; Hilleman, 1989; Porter, Glass, and Koff; Vermund). An HIV vaccine able to prevent or modify clinical disease and death would be very welcome, and very beneficial to vaccinated individuals, although perhaps with less direct benefit for the community (because infection would still occur and possibly be transmissible, although probably less efficiently). However, because of the long incubation period between HIV infection and clinical disease, it is impractical to wait for clinical endpoints of disease or mortality as indications of efficacy in the individual patient. Whether an HIV vaccine candidate will prevent infection or disease may not be known before it is tested, however, so both infection and disease endpoints (hopefully via surrogate markers) must be built into the first efficacy studies and decisions made about how to measure them and evaluate the results.[47]

Selection of endpoints will be influenced not only by the intended goal of vaccination, but also by the chosen vaccine candidate. Choice of endpoints has several ethical implications. If the goal is prevention of infection, the endpoint to be assessed should be a measure of infection. To be successful, a vaccine would have to permit no infection or at least cause a dampening of infection using one or more markers of infection. Tests currently in widespread use to determine if someone is infected measure anti-HIV antibody. It would be possible to distinguish antibody responses to natural infection from vaccine-induced antibody only if subunit vaccines are used (antibodies to the selected vaccine antigens versus antibody to all/most viral [wild-type] antigens could be noted on western blot analysis). If whole killed virus or live attenuated virus were used in a candidate vaccine, the vaccine would elicit antibody to all parts of the virus, and therefore vaccine-induced antibody responses would not be distinguishable from natural infection.[48] Other markers of infection might include virologic tests, such as the polymerase chain reaction (PCR), p24 antigen immunoassay, plasma viremia, or HIV culture. These tests used to detect virus itself are expensive, cumbersome, and not well standardized. Even if antibody tests are used as endpoints, some viral tests will probably be necessary to distinguish infection by strains of virus unprotected against, as well as to evaluate the vaccine candidate's effect on viral burden. Agreement on reliable measures of infection has yet to be achieved.

If the goal of vaccination is prevention of clinical disease or death, the chosen endpoints might be the development of clinically identifiable syndromes (such as certain opportunistic infections), surrogate markers of disease progression (such as measures of immune function or viral load), or even mortality. These are all problematic because of the considerable length of time required for clinical changes to occur, and the multiple influences affecting them. Clinical changes, for example opportunistic infections, typically occur only after the immune system is severely depressed, an average of ten years after infection (and with therapy or prophylaxis possible even longer). There is disagreement about the clinical significance of various "surrogate markers" of disease progression. Yet in order to evaluate efficacy within a reasonable time frame, surrogate markers of disease will need to be measured. More research on changes in surrogate markers that occur during natural infection will allow for a more meaningful measure of the influence of a vaccine.

A vaccine trial using clinical disease as an endpoint would need to include an adequately large randomized sample to allow for multiple influences; subjects might need to be followed for ten to twenty years or longer. If only clinical endpoints were chosen, considerable time might elapse during which the placebo group (if a reliable infection endpoint had been chosen and achieved) might have been protected from infection. Also, waiting for a clinical endpoint might deprive anyone who becomes infected (vaccinated or unvaccinated) from the benefits of early treatment. For all of these reasons, reliance on clinical endpoints alone is untenable, and selection of nonclinical endpoints is essential.

"It is important that we begin the process of developing a consensus on the acceptability of non-clinical markers of efficacy with the participation of a variety of interested and knowledgeable parties" (Petricciani et al., 1992, p. 1527). Besides consensus on the validity of nonclinical endpoints, reliable, available, and universally acceptable measures of the endpoint must be agreed upon. For example, if antibody response is chosen, there must be universally accepted standardized tests capable of distinguishing vaccine-induced antibody from antibody formed to wild virus *before* efficacy trials begin. Alternatively or in addition, tests providing direct evidence of viral infection that are doable, affordable, reliable, and standardized (and thus comparable) must be available. To be useful as endpoints, tests must be able to distinguish responses to vaccine from responses to infection in vaccinated individuals, as well as to distinguish responses to natural infection in vaccinated compared to unvaccinated individuals (placebo controls and nonparticipants). Results (vaccine responses versus responses to natural infection) not only must be distinguishable, but the distinction must be widely accepted, not only for the validity of results and comparisons with other studies, but also for the protection of the rights of study participants. Discrimination against persons who test positive for antibody to HIV is a tragic reality; therefore every effort must be made to reduce the possibilities for discrimination against those who develop HIV antibodies as a result of voluntary participation in a vaccine study. Official documentation of such participation is also essential.

Failure to reach consensus on standardized and available measures of efficacy could affect the validity of the research and therefore be harmful to the individual subjects and communities involved. A false negative result—for example, failing to achieve complete "sterilizing" immunity, or inappropriate selection of endpoints—might deprive populations of a potentially beneficial intervention (continuing the example, a vaccine may fail to prevent infection but be capable of preventing or modifying disease). A false positive result—for example, basing efficacy on inappropriate endpoints, accepting a low protective efficacy, or calculating efficacy in comparison to historical or unvaccinated controls—may jeopardize the conduct of further trials of more effective vaccines. In addition, studies which are not well planned and designed can result in the depletion of economic resources and available study sites and populations without any benefit, as well as erode public confidence and hinder vaccine development. The need to evaluate multiple vaccine candidates or approaches should be balanced with limited resources (funds and human volunteers).

Consensus about reliable, affordable, and standardized measures of efficacy endpoints is essential so that valid, generalizable, and useful results can be achieved in the most efficient manner, and thus the requirements of social beneficence can be adhered to (see Levine, Dubler, and Levine). The best approach might be to look for and evaluate an endpoint of *infection*, after establishing and agreeing upon reliable measures of infection capable of making the relevant distinctions. At the same time, plans should be in place to follow a substantial cohort of vaccinated and unvaccinated subjects, especially those who become infected, over a longer period of time in order to determine the effect of the vaccine on the development or course of clinical disease. This would involve the measurement over time of agreed-upon "surrogate markers" of disease, as well as evaluation of clinical manifestations, morbidity, and mortality. One scientist suggested comparing the entire cohort of vaccinated and unvaccinated groups at yearly intervals by screening for evidence of infection (using antibody and DNA PCR), measuring surrogate markers of disease (such as CD4+ cell count), assessing the presence and progress of clinical disease, and comparing mortality rates (Dr. Donald Burke, Institute of Medicine Roundtable Meeting, December 1992). Another suggestion is to follow the entire cohort for approximately three years after vaccination to evaluate the incidence of infection, and then follow the infected cohort for five to ten years longer to evaluate surrogate markers and clinical disease (Sten Vermund and Rod Hoff, Vaccine Branch, Division of AIDS, NIAID, personal communication, June 1993). Decisions about when or how often to measure these endpoints may vary. Because the spread and behavior of HIV are erratic, and exposure usually depends on voluntary behavior (which may be altered because of counseling provided as part of

p. 8. consensus statement #7). The consensus document further states: "No group should be categorically excluded, on the basis of age, gender, mental status, place of residence or incarceration, or other social or economic characteristics from access to clinical trials or other mechanisms of access to experimental therapies" (ibid., p. 14, consensus statement #30). The consensus group suggests that the burden of proof "should rest with those who would set narrow and strict exclusion criteria." Although the statement's focus is HIV drug trials, the same guidelines should also apply to vaccine trials. The sample selected should reflect the realities of the demographics of the disease (i.e., those at high risk) in the interests of good science and fairness and be chosen on the basis of potential benefits to the sample community compared to potential risks (as identified and perceived by the group) and a fair distribution of those benefits and burdens.

It is also unfair and exploitative to disproportionately expose certain groups to the burdens of research if the benefits will go elsewhere or be distributed more broadly. Guideline 10 of the 1993 CIOMS guidelines states: "Individuals or communities to be invited to be subjects of research should be selected in such a way that the burdens and benefits of the research will be equitably distributed. Special justification is required for inviting vulnerable individuals, and if they are selected, the means of protecting their rights and welfare must be particularly strictly applied" (p. 29). Historically, subjects and populations were sometimes selected for participation in vaccine research inappropriately (for example, captive populations, although at high risk of infectious diseases, were convenient, controllable, easier, etc.) and were often not the beneficiaries of the outcomes of the research in which they participated. The CIOMS guidelines say that justification of the involvement for "vulnerable" groups requires that investigators satisfy the review committees that (1) the research could not reasonably be carried out with less vulnerable subjects; (2) the research is intended to obtain knowledge that will lead to improved diagnosis, prevention, or treatment of diseases or health problems characteristic of or unique to the vulnerable class, either the actual subjects or other similarly situated members of the vulnerable class; (3) research subjects and other members of the class from which subjects are recruited will ordinarily be ensured of reasonable access to diagnostic, preventive, or therapeutic products that become available as a consequence of the research; (4) the risks attached to research not intended to benefit the individual subjects will be minimal, unless an ethical review committee authorizes a slight increase above minimal risk; and (5) when the prospective subjects are incompetent or otherwise substantially unable to give informed consent, their agreement will be supplemented by the proxy consent of their legal guardians or other duly authorized representatives (CIOMS, 1993, p. 30). U.S. regulations guiding human-subjects research include very similar requirements (45CFR.46.111 (3)). Hence, special justification and sometimes additional review are required for inclusion of certain groups (such as children, incompetent subjects, incarcerated persons), as is additional protection if they are included. Studies involving "captive" populations, such as prisoners or institutionalized persons, are rarely done today.

The issue of recruiting populations in developing countries as subjects in vaccine research is very controversial, especially with HIV. To avoid the appearance of "exporting" risks and exploiting populations in developing countries, a general consensus has been reached that HIV vaccines will first be tested through the first two phases in the country of the sponsor, and subsequently Phase I and II trials of promising candidates will be repeated in developing countries (CIOMS, 1993; FCCSET; USPHS, 1991). Phase III efficacy trials might then be done in both places in parallel. Some scientists believe that questions of efficacy may be answerable only in developing countries because of the higher incidence of infection found there.

Social justice requires that plans be made before research is conducted for the financing and utilization of a vaccine after it is proven to be effective. Smith and others state that populations should not be involved in the clinical testing of a vaccine if they will not be able to afford to buy and therefore utilize it after marketing, and ethically should be invited to participate only if there is a commitment to supply them with the vaccine (CIOMS, 1993; Esparza et al., 1991; Levine, Dubler, and Levine; Smith, Hayes, and Mulder). "From an ethical standpoint, to place a research burden on Third World countries and not make plans [to make the final product accessible] is unconscionable" (Larry Gostin, as quoted by J. Cohen, 1991, p. 1313). At a minimum, an effective vaccine should be provided to the placebo group, but a free or reasonably priced vaccine should also be provided to other members of the community or residents of the host country. From whom this commitment should come and how it will be managed are subjects of considerable debate. Several suggestions have been proposed, including a two-tiered pricing system in which developed countries pay more for the vaccine and thereby subsidize others; a patent exchange in which developers of an AIDS vaccine donate the patent to an international organization in exchange for extension of a patent on an existing drug; and financing and distribution of vaccines by the governments of industrialized countries or by an international organization, taking the vaccines out of the private sector altogether (ibid.).[50] No commitments or mechanisms have yet been established. In the model proposed in this book, the precise mechanisms of supply, financing, or subsidy of effective vaccines to the involved community would be worked out in community and national negotiations with the sponsors and investigators. If an agreement cannot be made that satisfies both parties, the research should not be conducted in that community (and/or country).

The sample selected for participation in an efficacy trial for an HIV vaccine should be chosen on the bases of scientific validity, generalizability, efficiency, respect for persons, beneficence, and justice, including fair distribution of the benefits and burdens of research and commitment to distributive justice of an effective vaccine. Practically speaking, this means selecting communities because of a high incidence and high risk of infection and a scientific compatibility between the prevalent strain(s) of virus and the vaccine candidate. Once the community is selected as a possible target population, community discussions and negotiations begin, first with the government and leaders of the community (usually preceded by approval at the national or regional level), and then with members of the community as a group (this is also discussed in chapter 3). Reasons for selecting that community, honest expectations of both short- and long-term benefits and risks of the proposed research to the community, the goals and methods of the proposed clinical trial(s), and the nature and extent of any commitment to provide primary health care, distribution of condoms or needles, compensation for injuries, and financing of marketed vaccines should all be presented to the community. Community members will then vote at a town meeting; if the majority of those present consent to the proposed research, then any seronegative member of that community who is interested, willing, and able to give informed consent should be considered eligible for participation.

It has been pointed out that the groups or communities at highest risk of HIV in the U.S. (and in many other places) are also groups which are "vulnerable" because of stigmatized behaviors, social or economic status, lack of adequate health care, etc. There could be accusations that these communities are being "used" as guinea pigs or disproportionately exploited in vaccine research. To run a scientifically useful study, the community must have a high incidence of HIV and of members at risk of acquiring HIV. If community members perceive themselves to be at risk and are willing as a group to participate in research aimed at preventing transmission of HIV, they will be the primary bearers of the burdens and benefits of vaccine research, and so justice may be adhered to. Those who conduct vaccine trials must be very careful to follow scientific and ethical principles and to respect the decisions of the community and its members.[51] Additionally, vaccine efficacy will need to be tested at multiple sites in order to assess generalizability and to test efficacy under variable conditions. Exploitation of certain communities will be minimized if the multiple sites chosen represent the spectrum of the demographics of infection and of viral strains (as the science dictates), and the communities themselves are empowered to decide whether or not they want to participate.

Size

In order to obtain an answer to efficacy, an adequately large sample should be derived from a population with a high enough seroincidence that there will be a reasonable expectation of exposure to infection in both the vaccinated and control groups (see Esparza et al., 1989; Gostin, 1987; Porter, Glass, and Koff; Vermund). The sample size must be large enough to allow for randomization, to account for the unpredictabilities of the spread of HIV, and to statistically balance the influences of counseling and education about risk reduction. Determination of sample size must also take into account dropout rates, compliance, cooperation, and changes in incidence over a considerable period of time. The sample size can be calculated based on estimated seroincidence in the population group, the endpoint to be evaluated, the duration of follow-up, and the desired efficacy of the vaccine (Esparza et al., 1991; Haynes, p. 1282; Sawyer, Katzenstein, and Quinnan; Smith, Hayes, and Mulder, p. S105).

The higher the seroincidence, the smaller the sample can be and still be able to demonstrate efficacy. Planners of HIV efficacy trials are in the process of identifying groups with high seroincidence as possible subject communities. Smith et al. caution that some populations with high incidence may be approaching "saturation" levels of infection which may serve to alter the risk of those who remain uninfected (p. S108). This is especially important if populations are selected now but may not be involved in vaccine testing for several years. "It may be difficult to identify a suitable sample population for HIV due to the rapidly changing epidemiology of the disease, one which may [probably will] change even during the course of a clinical trial" (Ellis, 1990, p. 402). A smaller sample with high seroincidence may reduce the costs and logistical difficulties of conducting a trial and make it easier to maintain high-quality field procedures and reliable data. It may also enhance the ability to provide attention and protection for each individual. However, these considerations must be balanced against the influences of behavioral change and other preventive strategies and of loss to follow-up. Even with significant seroincidence, it is estimated that each efficacy trial will require 500 to 2,000 volunteers (NIAID, 1993; Esparza et al., 1991, p. S161). Smith estimates that if a population with a seroincidence as low as 1 percent were used, more than 6,000 subjects would be needed for each trial (Smith, Hayes, and Mulder, p. S108).[52]

Composition
In addition to seroincidence (which determines the size and the power of the sample), other requirements of sample selection include stability and cooperation, and likelihood of benefit if the vaccine is found effective.

United States. Populations in the U.S. with relatively high seroincidence are primarily socially stigmatized groups often involved in activities which are not legally or socially sanctioned, such as IV drug users, prostitutes, and gay men. These sanctions may provide a disincentive to volunteering. Additionally, the majority of persons in the U.S. who are at high risk for HIV and could be recruited for participation in vaccine trials "have characteristics that warn us to scrutinize with care how and why they are selected, whether they are coerced, whether they are sincerely informed, whether they understand and are competent to consent, and whether the burdens and goods of society are being fairly distributed" (Novick, 1989, p. 125). Involving the community in discussions about the purpose and processes of research from the beginning, and giving community members important roles in the development, acceptance, and conduct of the research (through town meetings, community advisory boards, recruitment of local staff, community outreach educators, and other strategies), demonstrates respect for the community as a potential partner in the research endeavor.

The demographics of HIV in the U.S. are also changing; for example, the incidence in gay men has declined to less than 1 percent per year. Preparing sites by conducting research on other means of prevention may serve to reduce seroincidence even further. Other groups identified, including IV drug users and prostitutes, are traditionally harder to reach and believed to be less compliant. A balance will need to be sought between the requirements of high incidence and the often conflicting ones of stability and cooperation, in order to minimize loss to follow-up and maximize validity of results. Cooperation is especially crucial because of the proposed length of trial follow-up. Possible U.S. communities to be chosen for participation in HIV vaccine trials include those found in STD clinics, drug treatment facilities, community-based organizations serving homosexual men, prisons, and perhaps geographic communities (such as the East Bronx) with a high seroincidence, including through perinatal transmission (see more on this below).

Developing countries. Incidence rates in the general population of some developing countries may be high enough to permit an efficient evaluation of vaccine efficacy. A devastatingly high seroincidence, especially in some cities, may permit an earlier determination of efficacy, and perhaps with smaller numbers, than comparable studies in the U.S. Again, the issues of saturation, stability, cooperation, and justice must be considered. Certain groups, such as prostitutes, rural dwellers, and truck drivers, may be more difficult to reach than others. If stability and cooperation are carefully sought, and ethical issues attended to, selecting certain high-risk/high-seroincidence groups (such as female prostitutes) or stable groups (such as military personnel) may also be useful. Because of limited access to treatment or preventive services and a rapidly increasing incidence of HIV disease, participation in a vaccine trial may be seen as very beneficial by some villages or regions. This is especially true if the vaccine is effective, but also if the conduct of vaccine research is used as an opportunity for strengthening local capabilities for conducting research and/or delivering health care, as well as strengthening or introducing other HIV prevention efforts.

Investigators might be tempted, however, to conduct trials in developing countries because of reduced liability, less stringent restrictions and regulations, or less expense. Unfortunately, previous examples exist, including perhaps the testing of the first HIV vaccine in Zaire, and so distrust and suspicion about the motives and methods of foreign scientists and governments are common (Lurie et al.). The WHO/GPA, CIOMS, and others have recognized the potential for problems in international trials. As mentioned, it is generally agreed that Phase I and II studies of candidate vaccines will be done first in the country of origin of the vaccine, and then repeated in developing countries before Phase III vaccine trials are conducted, not only for reasons of fairness, but also because safety and immunogenicity may be different in different populations (e.g., the influences of nutritional status, other STDs, parasitic diseases, etc. on immune response) and because of strain variation. Consultation with, and approval by, government bodies in the potential host country should precede any decision about conducting trials in that area. Ethical review should be satisfied in both the sponsoring country and the country chosen to participate. The CIOMS guidelines specifically state:

> Externally sponsored studies undertaken in a host country, but initiated, financed, and sometimes wholly or partly carried out by an external national or international agency, with the collaboration or agreement of the authorities of the host country . . . [should fulfill] two ethical obligations: 1) The initiating agency should submit the protocol to ethical review in which the ethical standards should be no less exacting than they would be for a study carried out in the initiating country; 2) The ethical review committee in the host country should satisfy itself that the proposal meets its own ethical requirements. (1993, p. 43)

Subsequently, consultation with local community leaders, politicians, religious leaders, and media representatives in the target community would serve to begin the process of informing the people and enhance cooperation. "Town meetings" should be held with members of the community to inform them about the purposes and methods of the research and to invite their consent to participate as a community. The communities involved should be those with the greatest need for control and prevention of HIV—i.e., who not only are at risk but perceive themselves to be—and those who will ultimately utilize an effective vaccine.

Again, efficacy studies in any population will have to be lengthy. It may take a matter of years to reach endpoints, probably ten to fifteen years at minimum to know the true effects of the vaccine on clinical disease. Additional years may be needed to follow up for the possibility of rarer or long-term side effects, and years beyond that to measure the duration of any vaccine-induced protection. Postmarketing surveillance studies will be essential in this regard. The sample selected for participation in efficacy studies must be willing and able to comply with years of participation. Because of this, the requirements of the study cannot be too demanding, yet care must be taken to account for and evaluate all significant eventualities.[53] Input as to what demands the community would be willing and able to comply with will greatly enhance cooperation. An evaluation of the capabilities of available or newly established resources (laboratory, personnel, storage, data, etc.) will also help determine the specific requirements. Efforts to ensure compliance are essential, and may include reimbursement for expenses and coordination with other necessary health services. For example, some commentators have suggested providing transportation, child care, primary health care, or STD treatment (Novick, 1989; Phil Wilson, IOM Roundtable Meeting, December 1992). The rights of individual community members to give their individual consent or to refuse participation, to withdraw at any time without repercussions, to have their confidentiality protected, and to be informed of relevant information as it becomes available must also be respected.

SPECIAL POPULATIONS

Pregnant Women, Children, and Infants

Difficulties related to trial duration and costs, and unpredictability in measuring outcomes and proving efficacy have led some to suggest evaluating vaccine efficacy in the prevention of perinatal infection. By vaccinating infected pregnant women or neonates within the first few days after birth, researchers could evaluate a vaccine's ability to prevent infection within eighteen months or less of an infant's life. "In evaluating efficacy of an AIDS vaccine, trials in infants may be completed more rapidly because of the relatively short period between infection and disease onset that is characteristic of HIV infection in young children" (Sawyer, Katzenstein, and Quinnan, p. 41). Between 15 percent and 30 percent of children born to infected mothers are themselves infected, and more than half of those develop clinical disease within two years.[54]

The NIAID's Division of AIDS has two broad HIV vaccine-related goals within its pediatric agenda: postinfection vaccine therapy for HIV-infected children using the approaches being studied in adults, and prevention of perinatal transmission. Phase I trials of HIV vaccine candidates in infected pregnant women, infected children, and neonates born to infected mothers began in 1994 in the U.S. (Fast and Walker; NIAID, 1992). In addition to "holding the promise of preventing infection and disease in children, many researchers hope they may tease out the answer to the most baffling question facing AIDS vaccine developers: what must the immune system do to foil HIV?" (J. Cohen, 1992b, p. 1568).

Interestingly, rather than protesting the ethics of using these "vulnerable" children in vaccine testing (and before any efficacy data is available from adults), the more vocal have argued that it is unethical to exclude children and neonates because participation offers "a glimmer of hope for infected mothers and children" (ibid.). Given the threat of HIV to the children of the world, several authors suggest that there is a powerful ethical imperative to do research involving children (Ackerman, 1990; C. Levine, 1991b). Most of these discussions focus on children who are already infected and their need for effective therapies in the face of very few options. Recognizing a limit to that imperative, Carol Levine "cautions against allowing the current wave of optimism and enthusiasm for redressing the prior injustice of failing to consider the needs of pediatric HIV/AIDS patients to swamp the need to protect these vulnerable children" (1991b, p. 236). How, if at all, does this ethical imperative apply to vaccine trials? While children are the most susceptible to many other infectious diseases and the most likely to benefit from utilization of effective preventive vaccines (e.g., poliomyelitis, pertussis, measles, mumps, and others), HIV is primarily an infection of adults, transmitted by adult-type behaviors. The exception, of course, is infection of children born to infected mothers. Therefore, children as a group are not at high risk of acquiring HIV infection, are not likely to be the initial target group for an effective vaccine, and therefore should not be one of the first groups to bear the burdens of efficacy testing of preventive vaccines.

The Medical Research Council (MRC) of the United Kingdom concluded that including children and neonates in HIV vaccine studies was acceptable, yet including women of child-bearing potential was not (MRC, 1991). The MRC suggested limiting neonate inclusion to those "shown *not* to be infected (by their mothers) with HIV." These recommendations seem misguided in that uninfected babies as a group are the *least* likely to benefit from a preventive HIV vaccine, while women of child-bearing potential, especially female partners of infected men, female prostitutes, female intravenous drug users, and possibly health care workers, not only might benefit themselves (by avoiding infection or disease) from an effective vaccine, but also might reduce the possibility of transmission to their children.

The proposed studies which will affect neonates, either through vaccination of infected pregnant women or by vaccinating neonates born to infected mothers within a few days of birth, are troubling. In either case, 70 percent or more of the neonates exposed to the risks of the vaccine (including lifelong seropositivity) do not stand to benefit. In accordance with U.S. federal regulations, two considerations should be made before children are included in research:

1. Is the risk involved minimal or a "minor increase over minimal risk"? (45CFR.46, Subpart D). The risks for neonates in preventive HIV vaccine studies include the physical risks of immunotoxicity, which might be different in an immature immune system, as well as possible enhancement of disease (which, if it occurs, would occur only upon exposure to the virus, probably many years later) and the possibility of not being able to take another vaccine at a later date. Additionally, some of these children will become HIV positive and will begin a life vulnerable to the possible repercussions of that status (although it is hoped these can be minimized by careful policies to prove that it is vaccine-induced).[55] These risks taken together may represent more than a minor increase over minimal.

2. Does this research present an opportunity to understand, prevent, or alleviate a serious problem affecting the health and welfare of children? (45CFR.46, Subpart D). The answer to this question is clearly yes. If perinatal transmission could be effectively prevented, vertical spread of HIV might be eliminated. How do the conflicting answers to these two considerations balance? There is a danger of letting politics and a misunderstanding of the differences between treatment and preventive vaccines influence the decisions instead of good, meticulous science and careful attention to ethics.

U.S. federal regulations also limit the involvement of pregnant women as subjects to those research activities whose purpose is to meet the health needs of the mother and/or in which the risk to the fetus is minimal, and for which the informed consent of mother (and father where applicable) has been given (45CFR.46.207). If the proposed research aims to include evaluation of the vaccine as potentially therapeutic for the mother as well as potentially able to prevent transmission to the fetus, it may comply with the regulations if the risk to the fetus (especially the 70 percent who will not become infected anyway) is considered minimal. However, these are Phase I studies; therefore the aim is to evaluate safety.

The IRBs which reviewed these proposals found them acceptable. Cohen suggests that safety and immunogenicity data from adult trials, two state liability laws indemnifying companies making vaccines,[56] political muscle (a 1992 amendment to the NIH reauthorization bill mandated trials in pregnant women and children within a year), and further campaigning by influential players such as Dr. Robert Redfield (at Walter Reed, the principal investigator of Phase II therapeutic vaccine trials), Dr. Antonia Novella (the former U.S. surgeon general), and Dr. David Kessler (FDA commissioner) together created a sense of urgency in testing infected pregnant women and children with available vaccines (J. Cohen, 1992b, p. 1568). Certainly the political pressure is very influential (remember therapeutic gp160 trials). Yet there seems to be confusion between the goals of and justification for doing therapeutic vaccine trials versus those for prophylactic vaccines. There is clearly a great need for more pediatric HIV research in order to find effective treatment for HIV infected children and to find ways to prevent perinatal transmission.

Based on the risk/benefit analysis for neonates, it might be better to postpone Phase I trials of HIV vaccines in infected pregnant women or neonates until there is some evidence of efficacy in animals or other adults, i.e., some reason to believe that the vaccine candidates have a desirable effect.

The question has arisen whether potential or actual pregnancy should preclude participation in Phase III efficacy trials of a suitable HIV vaccine candidate (see, for example, NIAID, 1993a, p. 3; also FCCSET, p. 95). There are several reasons why it should not. First, the categorical exclusion of a whole class of people who are at risk of infection is discriminatory. Second, the Phase I and II trials described above, when complete, will provide safety data for pregnant women and neonates, so risk to the fetus, within limits, will be predictable. Third, there is potential benefit to women members of a community of participants, but perhaps more important, because women of child-bearing age are members of most high-risk communities which might be targeted (such as intravenous drug users, prostitutes, patients at STD clinics, geographic communities) and are clearly at risk, the community can be accurately represented and involved only if women are included. Again, each woman member of a consenting community would be invited to participate and asked to give her own informed consent. Potential dangers to the fetus if the woman were to become pregnant should be described, as should available methods of avoiding pregnancy.

Prisoners
U.S. federal regulations permit research involving prisoners only under limited conditions, including

on conditions particularly affecting prisoners as a class (for example vaccine trials on hepatitis which is much more prevalent in prisons than elsewhere . . .) provided that the study may proceed only after the Secretary has consulted with appropriate experts in penology, medicine, and ethics, and published notice, in the Federal Register, of his [her!] intent to approve such research; or

research on practices, both innovative and accepted, which have the intent and reasonable probability of improving the health or well-being of the subjects. (45CFR.46.306 (C) and (D))

Regulations also require that the IRB include a prisoner as a member; that there not be undue inducement to volunteer (in the form of living conditions, medical care, food, amenities, or earnings); that risks to prisoners be commensurate with those accepted by nonprison volunteers; that procedures for selection within the prison be fair; that information be presented in understandable language; that participation in research not influence parole; and that appropriate care be available to inmates during and after participation (45CFR.46.305 (1–7)). These regulations were based on recommendations of the National Commission on the Protection of Human Subjects of Biomedical and Behavioral Research (1983) at a time when research was considered risky, attention was focused on abuses, and there was a general lack of health care in prisons. The result has been the "virtual elimination of biomedical research activity in prisons and jails" (Dubler and Sidel, p. 185).

The HIV epidemic has challenged the basis for and interpretation of these recommendations and regulations. First, as described above and in chapter 2, the categorical exclusion of any group can be seen as discriminatory, especially if the benefits of participation in research are recognized. Second, HIV infection is particularly prevalent in prisons (for example, in the New York State prison system, 17.4 percent of inmates entering in 1988 were HIV-infected), and it is believed that this percentage will only increase (ibid., p. 181). At the same time, health and medical care in prisons are often woefully lacking. "[HIV-]infected inmates are shunned and often attacked, some have been killed. . . . Inmates with symptoms are left to suffer alone with inadequate or totally absent care" (ibid., p. 182). Third, behaviors which put one at risk of HIV infection are also prevalent in prisons. An estimated 40 to 80 percent of incarcerated persons admit to IV drug use (ibid., p. 181). Prison rape is common and is a "reflection of the violence and power struggles that characterize prison society. . . . This type of forced homosexuality is distinct from most homosexuality outside of prisons" (ibid., p. 182). However, because drug use and homosexual sex are prohibited in prisons (even though it is acknowledged that they occur), whether there is a high enough incidence of HIV infection to be able to test vaccine efficacy in prisons is unknown.[57]

The Medical Research Council of the United Kingdom recommends against inclusion of prisoners in vaccine trials as not "practicable" because of the problem of freely given informed consent, the lack of freedom to respond positively to counseling (condoms are not available, yet homosexual behavior is common), and the difficulty of maintaining confidentiality and the virtual inevitability of social discrimination (1991, p. 11, 2.18). Others have reached different conclusions on the involvement of prisoners, at least in HIV drug trials. "If effective safeguards can be designed to protect prisoners from harm or coercion, their participation in clinical trials might carry a fair risk to benefit ratio" (Novick, 1989, p. 127). Effective safeguards would need to include adequate protection of confidentiality and avoiding the situation where the only option for reasonable care is participation in the trial.

Prisoners as a group should not be excluded from HIV vaccine research and in fact may represent a population with high seroincidence and likelihood of benefit as a group. HIV vaccine research satisfies the qualifications specified in U.S. regulations because HIV is prevalent in prisons, and vaccines and risk-reductive counseling are practices which "intend to improve the health and well-being of subjects." It also satisfies Guideline 7 of the CIOMS Guidelines: "Prisoners with serious illness or *at risk of serious illness* should not arbitrarily be denied access to investigational drugs, *vaccines* or other agents that show promise of therapeutic or preventive benefit" (CIOMS, 1993, p. 24).[58] If, after appropriate approvals are obtained, the suggested process of community consultation and community consent is followed, the likelihood of discrimination within the prison or violence against prisoners who volunteer would be minimized, because the prison community as a whole would vote on whether to accept the research and would have some input into the specifics of the design. HIV vaccine research has potential benefits and risks for prisoners as a class or community of people and for the specific prison community that might participate, as well as for individual prisoners. The inmates in each prison would need the opportunity to weigh the potential risks and benefits and decide as a "community" whether they want to participate. If the prison community consents, then individual prisoners in the community would decide about their own participation.

There are practical problems which would have to be addressed to successfully conduct vaccine trials using prison communities. First, given the size of the population of a given prison, they most likely would have to consent to involvement in a multisite study. This factor complicates (actually limits) the negotiating power of each (sub)community if a standardized protocol is to be adhered to. Second, the duration of an HIV efficacy trial would probably be longer than the time of incarceration of a substantial proportion of prisoners; therefore, off-prison satellite sites for follow-up evaluations and a commitment from the individual prisoners to continue follow-up after being released would have to be established.

Intravenous Drug Users
Concern has been expressed that active intravenous drug users may not be competent to consent to participation in vaccine trials. Again, however, categorical exclusion of a group that stands to benefit is not justified. Special care will be necessary in providing information to persons actively using intravenous drugs, and efforts should be made to ensure that they, as

individuals and a community, understand the nature and the methods of the research. *Individuals* deemed incapable of understanding or voluntarily participating should not be included.

HOW SHOULD HIV VACCINE EFFICACY TRIALS BE DESIGNED AND CONDUCTED?

Recently, some have suggested that HIV vaccine efficacy should be tested within the context of broad-based prevention studies (Margaret Chesney, Anthony Fauci, and Phillip Wilson at the IOM Roundtable Meeting, December 1992; Jaffe, 1993; Snow, 1993) not limited to vaccine efficacy. The overarching goal is to determine the best (most reliable, most likely to be used, and most cost-effective) way to prevent HIV in at-risk persons and communities, and to control the spread of HIV in the population. For scientific rigor and to get the best and most useful answers, randomized controlled trials of preventive or behavioral interventions— studying, for example, the use of condoms, virucides, STD treatment, non-reusable needles, needle exchanges, reducing number of partners, etc.— could be planned and started now and ultimately include testing the efficacy of vaccine candidate(s). Research should be designed to evaluate means of preventing HIV attainable through counseling and behavior changes and to compare the efficacy of these to the efficacy of a vaccine, and not simply to try to determine vaccine efficacy in spite of ethical requirements to counsel and educate participants about risk reduction. Vaccine research conducted within a larger prevention research base communicates the message that learning about prevention is the goal and may thereby deflate accusations of exploitation, "using us for your vaccine," or "exporting risks" (domestically or internationally). Prevention research could be started without delay in target communities and serve as a public demonstration of the priority of preventing HIV, an opportunity to obtain valuable data on behaviors and the feasibility of conducting long-term research, an opportunity for educating the community about the goals and methods of research, including where vaccine research fits into the schema, and an opportunity for evaluating the community's cultural or social values and needs which might influence the design of nested vaccine studies and the range of commitments that should be considered.

Many behavioral change interventions to reduce the risk of HIV infection have already been implemented without the benefit of randomized controlled trials to demonstrate efficacy. Behavioral interventions may be perceived as harmless and effective, but some are expensive, some may actually increase high-risk behaviors, and it is not known how effective they are or what factors influence their effectiveness (Peterman and Sevgi). Because behavior is such a major factor in exposure to HIV, and behavior influences the ability to measure the efficacy of a vaccine, research done to better understand relevant behaviors in the community, as well as to get a handle on the influence of other methods of prevention on behavior and seroincidence (especially in the artificial conditions of clinical research), will also serve to facilitate the interpretation of data used to determine vaccine efficacy. It is also beneficial to the community and its individual members to determine the value and acceptability, and therefore the utilization, of other methods of prevention, given that an effective vaccine might be only 60 to 90 percent effective.

Studying other means of prevention of HIV can contribute to the success of determining vaccine efficacy (in ensuring cooperation and political will and a better understanding of behaviors) while fulfilling the obligations of beneficence and respect for research participants. As Dr. Harold Jaffe states, "We must hope for the best (that a vaccine will work), but plan for the worst (that it won't)" by doing everything possible to protect trial participants from infection (including those who receive placebo and nonefficacious vaccines) (Jaffe, p. S152). Evaluating preventive methods, which include, but are not limited to, vaccines, offers the best currently available protective intervention and serves to further knowledge in this area. Nonetheless, the possibility exists that the introduction or evaluation of other means of prevention may sufficiently reduce seroincidence in the target population that determination of vaccine efficacy is much more difficult or even impossible.

> The interests of beneficence mandate that individuals in all arms of an efficacy study be thoroughly counseled about HIV infection and high-risk behaviors. Participants must understand that they may not be receiving the candidate vaccine and that even if they do, the vaccine might not be protective. Participants . . . must understand the need to practice safer sex and other preventive behaviors even after immunization. The importance of reducing risk behaviors will persist because of the high probability that even a "successful" vaccine will be less than totally effective. In addition, uncertainties are likely to remain about the effectiveness of immunization against exposures to the virus by different routes of transmission and in different geographic areas. More behavioral research is necessary to better understand the potential effect HIV vaccine will have on behavioral change, so that strategies to encourage and sustain behavior change can be developed simultaneously with efficacy trials. The counseling message must be delivered or monitored by a party independent from the investigative team and must be regularly reinforced. *Although this complicates the evaluation of the candidate vaccine's efficacy, failure to provide basic information about risks for the sake of trial results denies the human dignity and welfare of participants, regarding them only as means to a research answer.* (FCCSET, p. 90; my emphasis)

A vaccine candidate would be added to an already established program of research. The most appropriate design for determining whether an HIV vaccine is effective in preventing infection or disease is a large, randomized, controlled, double-blind clinical trial. It would be useful (if consent could be obtained) to compare differences in the incidence of infection and disease not only between those who receive the experimental vaccine and those who receive placebo, but also to those who do not wish to participate in the vaccine part of the trial at all. (Previous vaccine studies have demonstrated a difference in disease incidence between placebo groups and nonvaccinated groups. See, for example, Clemens et al.)

The use of a placebo as a control is justified in the initial vaccine efficacy trials because no alternative preventive intervention other than counseling (which everyone will receive) is known. However, once a vaccine is shown to be even moderately effective, future candidates should be compared to it instead of to placebo. It is possible that those in the placebo group will ultimately have the same incidence of HIV infection (no differential in benefit) as vaccinees but with fewer risks, but it is also possible that more placebo recipients will become infected than vaccine recipients.

A double-blind design is desirable because subjects might practice more or less risk behavior if they knew they were in the vaccine group or the placebo group respectively, whereas the goal is to keep the two groups equivalent with respect to risk of exposure. Likewise, if investigators or the research staff knew which group the subject was in, assessment of behavior and side effects could differ, as well as the specifics of risk-reductive counseling. Concern has been expressed about the possibility of subjects unblinding or decoding themselves—for example, by obtaining the results of an antibody test which could distinguish vaccine from placebo. If a participant discovers s/he is in the vaccine group, s/he may feel more "protected," may actually increase risky behavior, and, by so doing, may bias the study (and the opposite if found to be on placebo). Decoding cannot be ignored or completely avoided. The best approach may be to recognize it up front and solicit the community's and each participant's commitment to the goals of the study which would be thwarted by decoding. At each visit when behavior is assessed, questions should be included to appraise the individual's knowledge or belief about which group he or she is in.

Even with a carefully designed randomized, blind, placebo-controlled study in which participants cooperate, vaccine efficacy will be very difficult to prove. There is a need for an adequate sample size, adequate duration, clearly defined endpoints, and satisfactory laboratory, clinical, and data-management staff and facilities. There must also be long-term commitment and support in the form of political will, resources, and services on the part of funders, sponsors, supporters, researchers, participants, and the community. If evaluation of other prevention strategies finds them to be more effective in reducing incidence than previously thought, vaccine efficacy will be harder to measure. Yet if the goal is truly to find the best way to reduce the incidence of HIV infection or disease, that would be an important and useful finding.

Scientists negotiating with a community must be clear about proposed endpoints, methods of measuring efficacy, methods of counseling for risk reduction, kinds of clinical and laboratory monitoring and standardization, compensation for inconvenience or injury, confidentiality, methods of confirming participation to reduce discrimination, etc. All of these issues must be attended to beforehand, communicated to the community of potential subjects, and agreed upon.

Careful planning of prevention trials must include several other things. First of all, there must be clinical facilities capable of handling large numbers, to screen and evaluate potential subjects, actually immunize vaccine participants, follow subjects for side effects, and evaluate endpoints of infection or disease over a long period of time. These clinical sites must be accessible to participants, have available support personnel, and have the capability for data collection, processing, and management.

Adequate and reliable laboratory facilities that can measure infection or disease endpoints and immune responses must also be available at field sites. Standardization and validation of laboratory tests should be done in advance. These facilities must be able to process and test the large number of samples collected during recruitment as well as during follow-up. Included are laboratory tests to screen and select potential subjects, monitor potential side effects of vaccines, evaluate vaccine-induced immune responses, and assess clinical and immunological parameters of infection and disease progression in vaccinated and unvaccinated subjects. Because tests of immune response are particularly complex and not standardized (as discussed in chapter 4), samples may have to be shipped to centralized reference labs for analysis, so facilities for appropriate storage, labeling, and shipping may also be needed.

Reliable and consistent methods of evaluating relevant behavior between visits should be incorporated into the assessment at each visit. It has been argued that in order to obtain more truthful answers regarding behaviors, behavioral assessments should be conducted by staff not involved in laboratory or clinical monitoring or in counseling (for example, Margaret Chesney suggested this at the December 1992 IOM Roundtable Meeting). Although separate staff for evaluating behavior and for clinical monitoring may seem to be the ideal, it may not always be possible or necessary. The establishment of a partnership in pursuit of a common goal (prevention of HIV) and an explicit expectation for all involved to commit to that goal may create an atmosphere of trust that permits more honest communication in both directions.

Appropriate referral mechanisms and facilities for counseling, treatment, and other needed services should be established for those found to be HIV-infected during the screening process and for those who become infected during the course of the study.

A long-term commitment at the national level, based on adequate political support and community participation at the local level, should be sought to make the conduct of trials possible (Esparza et al., 1991, p. S161, among others). As previously described, preparatory research should be conducted to facilitate the planning and conduct of large-scale prevention trials. This preparatory research might include epidemiological studies (of incidence, mobility of populations, incidence of potentially important concurrent conditions such as STDs, malnutrition, etc.), viral antigen isolation and characterization, social and behavioral studies (to evaluate methods which might motivate participation and/or compliance, to evaluate methods of risk-reduction counseling and of obtaining informed consent, and to evaluate current behavioral patterns), and pilot testing of the feasibility of vaccine-trial methodology (Esparza et al., 1991; also NIAID, 1993).

PROTECTING THE RIGHTS
OF PARTICIPANTS

INFORMED CONSENT

Each individual subject in vaccine-prevention research may in fact be asked to give his/her informed consent twice, once as a community member for the vaccine research to be conducted with that community, and again as an individual participant. Codes of research ethics (including Nuremberg, the Declaration of Helsinki, and CIOMS guidelines) and regulations in the U.S. and many other places around the world require the individual informed consent of each participant. Informed consent, based on respect for the person's autonomy and freedom to choose, is "consent given by a competent individual who has received the necessary information; who has adequately understood the information; and who, after considering the information, has arrived at a decision without having been subjected to coercion, undue influence or inducement, or intimidation" (CIOMS, p. 13). Consideration should be given then to the competence of potential subjects, what is the necessary information and how it should be presented in order to facilitate understanding, how adequate understanding will be determined, and what constitutes undue influence, inducement, or intimidation.

Competence

The general moral presumption that an adult is competent to make decisions is appropriate to the conduct of vaccine research (see Beauchamp and Childress, p. 82). Groups or communities of adults should be presumed competent to make collective decisions. The burden of proof should fall on the researcher or health care team who believes that a particular adult's competence is in question. (For example, active users of IV drugs should not be categorically considered incompetent, but their individual and collective ability to understand the research process and make voluntary decisions must be evaluated carefully.) For incompetent subjects, the consent of legally authorized representatives should be obtained.

Information

U.S. federal regulations provide a detailed list of the informational elements that must be included in obtaining the informed consent of a potential research subject (45CFR.46.116). These include:

> (1) a statement that the study involves research, an explanation of the purposes of the research and the expected duration of the subject's participation, a description of the procedures to be followed, and identification of any procedures which are experimental

For HIV prevention research, this should include an explanation of the goal of research as learning the value of experimental approaches to reduce the incidence of HIV infection in the community, including but not limited to the use of a vaccine. If a study is primarily designed to discover the correlates of immune protection, this should be so stated. Because the word *vaccine* is commonly associated with protection, some have suggested calling experimental vaccines something else (Snow, 1993). This seems unnecessary; however, the "experimental" should be emphasized so that false expectations are minimized. It should be very clear to all potential subjects that none of the methods under study may prevent HIV infection or disease completely, and that the goal is to find out how much and under what circumstances they do protect. Because of this, alternative methods of reducing risk will be suggested. Although primary endpoints of infection may be evaluated at three years or less, subjects should be aware and agree to be followed for ten years or more. They should also be aware that vaccine-induced immune responses may be permanent. A thorough description of methods (especially randomization, placebo controls, blinding) and procedures (laboratory monitoring, clinical monitoring, injection schedules, behavioral assessments, etc.) must be given, and those that are experimental must be identified. These descriptions must be in language understandable to the community of subjects.

(2) a description of any reasonably foreseeable risks or discomforts to the subject

This description should include possible risks to the individual and the community. The description should be of long- and short-term physical, psychological, and social risks and should include theoretical risks, those determined in Phase I and II studies, and the possibility of some unknown risks. For the individual, possible physical risks include local or systemic reactions to vaccine or placebo preparations, including local discomfort, allergic reactions, unknown neurological reactions, possibly other viral infections (depending on the vaccine preparation, e.g., vaccinia), or even HIV infection itself (in the case of live attenuated or whole inactivated viral vaccines); potential immunotoxicity or autoimmunity from vaccine antigens; possible future enhancement of disease; the possibility of not being able to take a future (perhaps more effective) vaccine; and the possibility of becoming infected (if a vaccine is only moderately effective, or if the subject is on placebo). Possible psychological risks include false expectations of protection from an investigational vaccine or a placebo leading to an increase in infection-exposing behaviors; the psychological burden associated with knowledge of HIV status in some cultures; the psychological burden of uncertainty; and the need to maintain safe behavior over a long period of time. Social risks include the potential for discrimination because of participation in the research itself and because of vaccine-induced seropositivity. All measures designed to minimize associated risks should also be described. For example, participants should be informed about the availability of antibody tests capable of distinguishing vaccine-induced antibody from natural anti-body, as well as how participation in the vaccine trial will be documented and confirmed.[59]

As argued earlier, potential short- and long-term risks to the community of which the subject is a member should also be considered and the community and its individual members informed of these risks. They in-clude the potential, again based on false expectations, for a general increase of risky behavior which might negate or minimize decreases in incidence caused by the vaccine (especially if the vaccine is only moderately effective) or other preventive interventions; the potential for vaccine-induced injury or harm or for finding the vaccine worthless or ineffective, either of which could have a negative impact on vaccine availability (because of liability con-cerns), on confidence in vaccines in general, and on confidence in clinical research (and the feasibility of testing future HIV vaccines or therapies), the potential for diverting or wasting limited resources; and the possibility of discrimination against the entire community (because of a perception that only high-risk persons or communities are included).

(3) a description of any benefits to the subject or to others which may reason-ably be expected from the research

It should be very clear to potential subjects that any direct benefit will go primarily to the community. If the vaccine is proven effective and is made available and widely utilized by the community, the incidence and thus transmission of HIV infection or disease in the community will be reduced. Other communities will also ultimately benefit from the results of this re-search. Individual subjects might also benefit, if they are in the vaccine group, receive a reasonably effective vaccine that protects against the rele-vant strain and route of infection, and are exposed to HIV infection at some time. Uncertainty about vaccine benefit and the probability that effectiveness will, at best, be less than 100 percent must be stressed. Additionally, partici-pants should be informed of potential community benefit through a commitment from the researchers to infrastructure building, training, labor-atory or clinical support or equipment, and the introduction and evaluation of other means of prevention of HIV (some of which will also be under study). If it is decided that certain other benefits, such as access to primary medical care, treatment of STDs, treatment of addiction, or the use of an active "placebo" (e.g., HBV vaccine), will also be provided, potential sub-jects should be so informed. Also included should be an explanation of arrangements made to subsidize or provide vaccine to the community after the trial.

(4) a disclosure of appropriate alternative procedures or courses of treatment, if any, that might be advantageous to the subject

As previously described, each individual participant should be carefully educated about other methods of reducing the risk of HIV infection. Avail-able data on the effectiveness of each of the methods described should also be provided. Methods which are being evaluated as part of the prevention study should be clearly described. Participants should also be instructed to consistently practice other risk-reductive behaviors during (and after) vaccine trials and informed that they will be counseled to do so throughout the trial and be questioned about their practices and behaviors at study visits.

(5) a statement describing the extent, if any, to which confidentiality of records identifying the subject will be maintained

Careful records which identify the participants in vaccine research and follow them over considerable periods of time will need to be kept. These records will contain sensitive information about behavior and exposure to risk. Investigators should describe to potential subjects where and how these records will be kept and who will have access to them. Some identifiable data will be sent to centralized laboratories or data-management facilities. The limits of the investigators' ability to protect these data should be carefully described to the subject. The possibility of discrimination because of participation in the research should be presented, and efforts to minimize the possibility of breaches of confidentiality and discrimination should be described. Community involvement and suggestions may help to minimize discrimination.

Some people will be identified as being HIV-infected during screening, and some will become infected during the course of the study. How this information will be dealt with will depend on the reporting requirements of the jurisdiction (some require reporting of infected persons, some require partner notification, etc.). Options and limitations should be presented to the community, and a decision made as to the processes of reporting and referral. These decisions and procedures should be adequately described to potential individual subjects before they consent.

(6) for research involving more than minimal risk, an explanation as to whether any compensation and an explanation as to whether any medical treatments are available if injury occurs and if so, what they consist of, or where further information may be obtained

The conditions under which compensation for alleged vaccine-induced injury will be provided should be delineated, including what criteria will be followed for determining if it is vaccine-induced, what kind of compensation will be available (medical care, lost wages, disability, etc.), and how the amount will be determined. Whether medical care will be provided, merely be compensated for, or neither should be covered, as should a description of other recourse which the subject may have (for example, tort claims or national compensation schemes).[60]

The CIOMS "International Ethical Guidelines for Biomedical Research Involving Human Subjects" (1993) state that "research subjects who suffer physical injury as a result of their participation are entitled to such financial or other assistance as would compensate them equitably for any temporary or permanent impairment or disability. In the case of death, their dependents are entitled to material compensation. The right to compensation may not be waived" (Guideline 13). These guidelines impose a stronger requirement to compensate for research-induced injury than the U.S. federal regulations, which require only informing potential subjects of the extent to which compensation will be provided, if at all. Interestingly, the commentary accompanying Guideline 13 (CIOMS) distinguishes compensation for injury that results from procedures which are done *solely* for research from those "expected or foreseen adverse reactions from investigational therapies or other procedures performed to diagnose or prevent disease" (CIOMS, 1993, p. 37), suggesting that justice demands compensation only for the former. The commentary further states that if it is unclear whether a procedure is performed primarily for research or for therapeutic purposes, the ethical review committee will decide what should be compensated for. Since, as argued in chapter 3, vaccine research is in a gray zone between therapeutic and nontherapeutic research, compensation for vaccine-induced injuries might legitimately be decided by ethical review committees (and in that case may be decided differently in different places). U.S. sponsors and trial designers should decide what injuries they can compensate for and how, and include this information in community negotiations, the review process, and the informed-consent process.[61] For international trials, review committees at the national level should decide initially if proposed compensation schemes are acceptable before community and individual acceptance is sought.

> (7) an explanation of whom to contact for answers to pertinent questions about the research and the research subjects' rights, and whom to contact in the event of a research-related injury

Communities and individual participants should be informed of who the sponsors and the principal investigators of the study are, and given ways to contact them if necessary. Participants should also be informed of the availability of local staff and community leaders involved in the conduct of the study who can answer questions and address their concerns, as well as the composition of the community advisory board and the existence of any community outreach workers. These individuals should be introduced at the town meetings. Also presented should be the existence and role of any oversight committees (including the IRB which approved the protocol) and the data and safety monitoring board (DSMB).

> (8) a statement that participation is voluntary, refusal to participate will involve no penalty or loss of benefits to which the subject is otherwise entitled, and the subject may discontinue participation at any time without penalty or loss of benefits to which the subject is otherwise entitled

Affirmation that each subject's participation is voluntary and refusal is not subject to penalty is extremely important, especially after the community of which the individual is a member has given its collective consent to conduct research (because it is possible that an individual will consent to the conduct of research in his/her community but not want to participate personally). Individuals must be informed that although they are free to withdraw from the research at any time, they may be permanently left with the immune changes and seropositivity caused by the vaccine.

Understanding

Because of the volume and complexity of the information provided, it is important that the individual's understanding of the information be evaluated and steps be taken to make it as complete as possible. In some of the early Phase I HIV vaccine trials in the U.S., written tests were administered to confirm that potential subjects had a basic understanding of the research before consenting. However, in the context of poverty and illiteracy, which are realities in a significant proportion of the target communities throughout the world, different ways of obtaining and assessing understanding must be sought. Community meetings, written and pictorial information, radio spots, and evaluating recall may all be helpful. The creative application of videos might be a useful mechanism. The identification and involvement of trusted community leaders or figures, such as community outreach workers, in providing and clarifying information and in making information culturally meaningful is crucial. Active involvement of community or host country scientists should be solicited. Staff involved in the day-to-day operations of the study should, when possible, be recruited from the community and be available to help with the ongoing provision and clarification of information. Consent for participation should not be accepted from individuals who do not understand the information after appropriate attempts have been made to facilitate understanding (this includes an understanding of the purposes and methods of research, as well as realistic expectations).

Voluntariness

The final and in some ways most difficult consideration in the process of informed consent is ensuring that the individual's consent is voluntary and free of coercion and undue inducement. As previously discussed, all decisions are made in the context of competing influences, so the trick is determining when other influences are controlling and voluntariness is compromised. The proposed process of community negotiation and consent may create a situation in which individuals feel *more* compelled to participate because their community approved. "Perhaps the most serious potential problem is that the consultation process may work to diminish rather than enhance participants' perceived freedom to raise questions about the research, consider the alternatives thoughtfully, and choose among them" (Melton et al., p. 577), referred to by Melton and colleagues as "groupthink." Certain steps can be taken to minimize this possibility.[62] Again, reinforcing and protecting each *individual's* right to volunteer or refuse to participate is essential.

Cultural values may also complicate or compromise an individual's ability to freely "volunteer" (for example, adolescents and women in some parts of the world). But although individuals must provide their own individualized consent, this does not preclude consultation with family members, friends, tribal or community leaders, or others.

Undue inducement to participate may occur if material goods (money, health care, treatment of STDs or drug addiction, HBV vaccine, condoms, better living conditions, etc.) are offered that cannot be obtained or are very difficult to obtain outside of the study. "Benefits" should be chosen that are sustainable after the research is over, that serve to improve local capabilities for doing research or delivering health care. However, strengthening the research infrastructure (for example, through technology transfer and capacity building) "should not be thought of as foreign assistance, [but as] a necessary step to ensure successful trial completion" (FCCSET, p. 70). Compensation for transportation, child care, and other expenses incurred because of trial visits is also legitimate. Efforts to make participation as convenient as possible, through mobile units, outreach programs, and the like, may minimize the need for extensive compensation for inconvenience and also help to ensure compliance. Achieving a balance between offering compensation and extra benefits to trial participants and avoiding coercion or undue inducement is essential, but will not be accomplished easily. It should be remembered that some individuals will participate solely for altruistic motives or to help their communities (for example, see Rida, Meier, and Stevens), while others will refuse no matter what is offered (see Snow, 1993). Ethical review at the national and local (IRB) levels, as well as community negotiation and input about the particulars of compensation to subjects will help to avoid the reality or perception of coercion, undue inducement, and/or exploitation.

> Subjects may be paid for inconvenience and time spent, and should be reimbursed for expenses incurred, in connection with their participation in research; they may also receive free medical services. However, the payments should not be so large or the medical services so extensive as to induce prospective subjects to consent to participate in research against their better judgement ("undue inducement"). All payments, reimbursements, and services to be provided to research subjects should be approved by an ethical review committee. (CIOMS, 1993, Guideline 4)

The CIOMS believes that the ethical review committee is the best judge of what is reasonable and what is "undue" influence, especially because these determinations may vary individually and also by culture and tradition. The input of the community can only strengthen this analysis.

MINIMIZING RISK

Although informed consent is the minimally necessary condition for respecting the rights of individual participants, alone it is insufficient to protect subjects' rights. Independent ethical review of all research proposals, and efforts to minimize predictable risk as much as possible are also essential. Two important considerations in minimizing risk to participants in HIV vaccine trials are efforts to reduce possible discrimination and mechanisms for monitoring data and terminating trials.

Vaccine-Induced Seropositivity and Discrimination

As already pointed out, many participants in vaccine trials for HIV will become (by standard tests) antibody-positive for HIV. Although subjects will have been informed of the probability of vaccine-induced seropositivity and the associated potential for discrimination because of it, other means of minimizing the risk of such discrimination are called for. While some HIV Phase I vaccine trials have provided participants with documentation of participation and toll-free numbers for obtaining confirmation of participation, such documentation has been insufficient to protect individuals from discrimination by the military, insurance companies, employers, and others. Illustrative examples have been provided by the staff of the Division of AIDS, NIAID.

In one case, a visiting professor at a U.S. university with an AIDS Vaccine Evaluation Unit volunteered as a low-risk participant in Phase I vaccine evaluation. Seroconversion occurred (Jack Killen, Special Assistant to the Director, NIAID, personal communication, April 1993). This individual was accepted for a faculty position at the university but was denied a visa by the U.S. Immigration and Naturalization Service (INS) because of his seropositivity. "The INS will not accept the volunteer's offer of letters and information from the NIH nor accept that the volunteer is not infected" (NIAID network communication). Letters from the principal investigators of the study were also not accepted by the INS. Amazingly, the only advice the INS was willing to accept was that of the Centers for Disease Control (CDC) branch with responsibility for Visa Medical Activities. Although the CDC, like the NIH, is part of the U.S. Public Health Service, the people in that branch were not "in the HIV/AIDS loop" and were unaware of the existence of, or implications of, vaccine-induced seropositivity. This particular case was finally resolved by high-level discussions between NIAID and CDC personnel and subsequent CDC communication with the INS. However, concern was expressed by the involved CDC official that the Senate bill designed to prevent HIV-infected persons from entering the U.S. states as a criterion "evidence of HIV infection," and this clause may be a problem for future visa applications. One NIAID official responded by suggesting non–U.S. citizen status as an exclusion criterion for future vaccine trials. This story underscores how difficult it can be for individuals to convince others that they are seropositive because of vaccine, even with documentation. It is also ironic that government officials would not accept the affidavits of other government officials.

Resolution of this and other cases has been achieved only through intervention by authorities in the Division of AIDS, NIAID. Yet, to date, about 1,500 individuals have participated in vaccine trials, and not all have seroconverted (at the lowest doses in some of the Phase I trials, antibody was not detectable). The prospect of intervening on an individual basis, at the time of discrimination, for the lifetimes of tens of thousands of volunteers all over the world is overwhelming, and the possibility of successful resolution in most cases is negligible. Serious efforts to widely publicize the conduct of large vaccine efficacy trials, the resultant seropositivity caused by the vaccine, and information about how to distinguish this from natural infection are absolutely essential but will not be enough. Discussions and explanations with health care personnel, insurance companies, the military, the INS, and others may also help, as will continued efforts at minimizing discrimination against infected persons (including, for example, changing the immigration laws). Official documentation of participation, easy and permanent access to registries (which also strive to maintain confidentiality) of participants, and advocates at the government level to intervene when necessary may be the best that can be done.

Data and Safety Monitoring
In order to minimize risks, adequate monitoring of data during the trial is essential. A data and safety monitoring board (DSMB) should be appointed for vaccine efficacy trials to assess safety data and achievement of endpoints. The DSMB should consist of vaccine experts, clinicians, biostatisticians, ethicists, and community representatives. The board would monitor data on a regular basis and make recommendations to the sponsors and investigators about continuing, modifying, or terminating the study, or about amending the informed consent process or form(s) (CIOMS, 1993, p. 40). Clear guidelines for stopping the trial should be established prior to initiating the study and adhered to by the DSMB. The board should also be given the authority to stop the trial early based on unanticipated or unacceptable adverse events, early demonstration of vaccine efficacy, lack of power to detect efficacy levels, the availability of scientific results from other vaccine trials, or external events such as war in the host country (Rida, Meier, and Stevens, p. 5). For collaborative trials, especially those that involve communities in different countries, a joint DSMB or WHO committee may fulfill this important role (FCCSET).

THE PROCESS OF DECISION MAKING AND REVIEW

Because of the complexity of conducting HIV vaccine research and the potential impact on individuals, communities, and the world, thoughtful and thorough reflection, review, and planning should occur at multiple levels and continue throughout the proposal, implementation, and evaluation stages of research.

RESEARCH PRIORITY SETTING

First, there should be a national body which sets priorities for research by considering public health needs, scientific possibilities, competition for resources, and community input. Presumably, this national body would select

HIV vaccine research as a priority. One could argue that in the U.S. this function is performed by Congress. Congress certainly has access to information about needs and possibilities and community interests, and votes on an annual basis to authorize and appropriate moneys for certain programs of research through the NIH and other agencies. Unfortunately, members of Congress are not always impartial in their setting of priorities and are often swayed by powerful lobby forces and/or by the desire to be reelected. Also, they approve or disapprove programs of research presented to them by agencies which are also motivated by influences other than need and public interest. "Politics and profits are as likely as science to impede the development of a vaccine. Many drug companies are reluctant to invest in research that might backfire dramatically and infect healthy people" (Arno and Feiden, pp. 20, 21). The USPHS, the DOD, other agencies, and their subcomponents also set priorities for research. Mechanisms for public input are almost nonexistent.

SCIENTIFIC STEERING COMMITTEE

Second, there should be careful scientific review of data generated, of candidate vaccines selected, and of the proposed methods and pace of research. This scientific review, perhaps by a "scientific steering committee," should be performed by a group composed of scientists (from both the public and private sectors, including representatives of vaccine manufacturers), epidemiologists (and/or clinical trial experts), clinicians, and community representatives from around the country. They should have access to data being generated in the public and private sectors in order to have a complete picture of the science and to make comparisons. This group would make recommendations to the sponsors and funders of research as well as to investigators. Scientifically sound guidelines for preclinical and clinical research of vaccines would be generated from this group. In the U.S., the NIAID Working Group on Vaccines, the AIDS Research Advisory Council, and the ad hoc groups formed by the NIAID are performing this function. The IOM Roundtable, the FCCSET subcommittee, and others are contributing to critical scientific review at the national level. Internationally, the WHO/GPA Vaccine Steering Committee is reviewing the science and making recommendations on the conduct of research in many countries around the world, as well as working with national scientific bodies in several countries.

NATIONAL APPROVAL

If consistent with national priorities for research and recommended scientifically, the next step is approval at the national level for the conduct of clinical research on preventive HIV vaccines in specific populations. National approval is especially important for externally sponsored research. As one official from the Thai Ministry of Health said, "[Even in international collaborative trials] the national sovereignty of each country must be respected. . . . HIV vaccine trials should only be conducted after obtaining the required official approval from appropriate national authorities" (Kunasol,

p. S135). Usually the ministry of health or a component of it will be the appropriate channel to gain official national approval for conducting vaccine trials. Many countries have established a national plan for research and control of HIV, often in conjunction with the WHO/GPA. Proposed research should be compatible with these plans.

REVIEW OF ETHICAL ISSUES
Once there is national approval to conduct vaccine research, there should be national review of the ethical and scientific merits of the proposed research. Some have suggested that a scientific steering committee or the equivalent should be responsible for both scientific integrity and adherence to sound ethical practice (e.g., Medical Research Council, p. 19). The CIOMS states that "scientific and ethical review cannot be clearly separated; scientifically unsound research on human subjects is *ipso facto* unethical in that it may expose subjects to risk or inconvenience to no purpose. Normally, therefore, ethical review committees consider both the scientific and ethical aspects of proposed research . . . and operate most effectively at the national level" (1993, p. 38). Although ethical review must be undertaken by a committee with at least some members who understand the science, there are two distinct functions to accomplish which could conceivably be achieved by one or two committees, depending on the composition and the purview of each. One function is critical review of the science and recommendations for future preclinical research and scientifically justified and valid clinical research (as described above for a scientific steering committee). The other function is, given the direction of the science, how the required human-subjects research can be carried out most in accordance with ethical principles and respect for the individuals, communities, and societies in which it will be conducted. A national ethics advisory board or analogous body might be responsible for the second function for many different kinds of research. The WHO/GPA has provided some guidance to the international community on criteria for the ethical conduct of clinical trials for HIV vaccines, as has the CIOMS through published general guidelines for the ethical conduct of research. Government bodies have published specific recommendations on the ethical conduct of AIDS vaccine trials (MRC, 1991).

There is currently no public forum in the U.S. which can consider and provide ethical guidance at the national level in the case of research with inherent or unique complexities. Resolution of problems faced in the clinical testing of HIV vaccine candidates might be enhanced if there were a central, independent body representing diverse segments of the community (policy-makers, scientists, potential subjects, ethicists, public health professionals, community representatives, and others) to address them. The role of such a body would not be to consider the specifics of any given research protocol (this is the purview of local IRBs) but rather to address issues and provide recommendations for a group of related studies with a common goal (such as a preventive HIV vaccine). This group could also be very helpful in addressing issues of clinical research involving gene therapy, fetal research, and many others. The creation of a standing ethics advisory board or similar body to reflect on and discuss these issues publicly and to make recommendations to the Department of Health and Human Services is a reasonable way to fill this void. "A standing Ethics Advisory Board that holds public hearings and focuses the best available ethical thinking on problems raised by ever advancing technology offers the best hope of matching high quality ethical policies with excellent science" (letter from John Fletcher and Charles McCarthy to Senator Hatfield and staff, 1993). Communities presented with the option of participating in research could appeal to this body for guidance. Alternatively, ethicists and persons familiar with the application of ethical guidelines to clinical research should be essential participants in federally sponsored and international working groups and scientific steering committees addressing HIV vaccines; as consultants to pharmaceutical or biotechnology firms involved in the clinical research of candidate vaccines; as members of local IRBs; and as members of data safety and monitoring boards.

COMMUNITY REVIEW AND APPROVAL

In adherence to the scientific and ethical recommendations and guidance, and after obtaining approval to proceed at the national level, investigator/sponsor teams should approach target communities. First, meetings should be held with official community leaders and scientists. With their help and the help of informal leaders and local media representatives, community meetings or "town meetings" should be held. The purpose of these meetings is to enlist the community and potential participants as partners in solving a difficult community problem. At the town meetings, investigators should present the proposed aims and methods of research in order to inform and educate the community and solicit input. Ultimately— probably after several community meetings, press coverage, and other information distribution—the consent of the community to conduct proposed vaccine research will be sought. Consent should be obtained through voting at the community meetings, as well as through a general campaign soliciting community feedback (for example, through a local office or telephone number). An advisory board or working group representative of the community should be created to discuss and negotiate the specifics of protocol design and methods. "Perhaps the strongest argument for community consultation is that it in fact increases procedural justice and embodies respect for the personhood of potential recipients" (Melton et al., p. 576).

LOCAL IRB REVIEW AND APPROVAL

The next step would be submitting the written research protocol(s) (which have been fashioned by the investigator/sponsor and the community advisory board) to the local IRB. "The design and performance of each experimental procedure involving human subjects should be clearly formulated in an experimental protocol which should be transmitted for their consideration, comment, and guidance to a specially appointed committee independent of the investigator and the sponsor" (Helsinki, 1989). The IRB performs its usual mission of reviewing the protocol(s) to ensure that there is a favorable risk/benefit ratio, that the rights of participants will be protected, and that subject selection is equitable. The IRB should have access to information about the deliberations and decisions of the community and the community advisory board. For externally sponsored research, IRBs in both the sponsoring and the host country should review and approve the research.

INDIVIDUAL PARTICIPANTS' REVIEW AND CONSENT

After the IRB approves the research protocol(s), individual participants should be recruited, informed, and screened. If they are interested and willing and able to give informed consent (i.e., competent to make decisions, fully informed, understand the information, and can voluntarily agree), they may be entered into the study.

DATA AND SAFETY MONITORING BOARD

As stated, a data and safety monitoring board (DSMB) should be created before the initiation of an approved clinical trial. The DSMB will meet periodically to monitor the data generated from the trial and to make recommendations to the investigators and sponsors. The board also has the power to decide what and when information obtained from the trial (or from other related trials) should be given to investigators and subjects.

Once individual informed consent is obtained and a person is enrolled in the clinical trial, counseling and clinical, laboratory, and behavioral evaluation will begin. Injections will be given according to the specific protocol schedule, and follow-up visits will be scheduled. During the trial, information should be provided to individual participants as indicated. Additionally, community town meetings should be held at regular intervals (every six or twelve months at a minimum) in order to update the community, obtain feedback, and enhance ongoing support and commitment.

CHAPTER SIX

▲
—————————————————————————————————
▼

Summary

The expanding global impact of the HIV epidemic has led to widespread acknowledgment of the need for an effective method of preventing and controlling HIV infection. Vaccines have been effective at controlling many viral infections in the past. Although HIV behaves differently than most other human viruses, control of HIV infection through a vaccine appears scientifically possible despite formidable scientific obstacles.

Applying the simple equation of addressing a great public health need with a traditional public health solution is complicated in the case of HIV. HIV infection has been associated in the minds of many with social deviance, and its impact has been concentrated in socially isolated populations; consequently, public and private responses to the problem have varied. Some argue against the need for and commitment of resources to develop an effective vaccine. Primarily a sexually transmitted disease, HIV infection, they argue, can be prevented by the avoidance of high-risk behaviors. But the type of behaviors that put one at risk of acquiring this disease are very personal and highly resistant to change. Additionally, the risk of infection is sometimes not associated with voluntary behavior at all.

Developing an effective vaccine against HIV (or any disease) is a long and complex process. First, basic research is necessary to understand the behavior of the virus itself and the resulting reactions of the human immune system. This is a crucial step, since vaccines work by manipulating or mimicking natural protective immune responses. Determining safe and productive methods of delivering and producing a vaccine is also necessary.

Vaccines are then tested in *in vitro* or animal models to evaluate their safety, immunogenicity, and protective ability before clinical studies are undertaken in human beings. Human testing of an experimental vaccine is the only decisive method for determining its usefulness. In order to find a safe and protective HIV vaccine, testing in humans is essential.

Clinical testing of vaccines occurs in three sequential phases involving human subjects: First a vaccine's safety is determined, then its immunogenicity, and finally its effectiveness at providing protection from infection or disease. Although understood as essential, the clinical testing of an HIV vaccine is fraught with many concerns. Inadequate understanding of immune responses to infection, the lack of an appropriate animal model, antigenic variation, and the newness of many immunological measurements have all hampered progress toward evaluation of safety and immune responses in human beings. Concern about safety (in the face of a dangerous and puzzling virus) and liability (in the face of such a public and controversial disease) in the development of an HIV vaccine have been countered by intense political pressure and scientific competition. The ethical, legal, social, and political concerns that accompany all clinical research have emerged as particularly acute and problematic in the case of HIV.

Many have turned to available guidance and tradition to find solutions to the dilemmas of conducting HIV research. Clinical trial methodology, regulations guiding the development and approval of drugs, and ethical guidelines concerning the conduct of human-subjects research have all been recently reevaluated and in some cases criticized and revised. Spurred in part by the HIV epidemic, clinical research is being looked at in a new light. Many have claimed that participation in research is a benefit, and have demanded a voice in the decision making and the process. Most of this attention has been directed to guidelines, regulations, and methods of clinically testing drugs, however, so the question of whether and how these discussions and revisions pertain to vaccine research has only begun to receive attention.

For human-subjects research with vaccines to be justifiable, it must have the potential for social benefit through the generation of useful/practical knowledge. But, as in all research, social benefit is only the minimally necessary condition for research, and must be balanced by respect for participants, benefit (or at least no harm) to participants, and justice. Since the goal of a vaccine is reduction of transmission and infection in a community through protecting individuals and reducing the reservoir of infection, the primary participant and beneficiary of vaccine research is the community. Individuals benefit as members of the community, and personally if protected upon future exposure to the infection. This kind of research is distinct from that in which the primary participant and potential beneficiary is the individual, or society at large. This book has recommended the recognition and addition of a third category of legitimate research in which the client and principal beneficiary is the community. Consequently, the social benefits of research would need to be balanced by respect for the community and its members, benefit to the community, and equity (both within the community and between communities). Respect for the community and its members entails more than respecting individual or group rights, and includes respect for the communal nature of individuals and their capacity and willingness to work in solidarity with others. The ethical conduct of research in which the primary participant and beneficiary is the community would require a three-way partnership between the investigators, the community, and the members of the community. Partners would be working together to achieve a common goal to satisfy mutual interests of importance to all of them.

In the specific case of HIV, these concepts would require that the communities that stand to benefit most from an HIV vaccine be invited to participate as partners in the endeavor. Since the goal is prevention of infection, the research agenda should be broader than just evaluation of a vaccine and include evaluation of other means of preventing or controlling HIV. With scientific possibilities in hand and the necessary national approvals in place, investigators should establish a partnership with target high-risk communities, presenting them with the research goals, methods, uncertainties, and logistics and seeking their collective consent to the research. Once a community has understood the proposed research and consented to participate, negotiations about the specifics of the conduct of research would occur through the establishment of a community advisory board. Detailed and specific protocols would then be submitted to a local IRB for approval, and presented to individual members of the community for consideration. Individuals would be free to participate or not and to withdraw at any time, and they would be treated fairly and with respect.

Although in some regards a radical departure from the way in which vaccine research is generally undertaken, the proposed partnership with involved communities and its members will serve to ethically justify the conduct of HIV vaccine research as well as to facilitate the practicalities of its conduct. Empowering the involved communities and their members as partners not only demonstrates respect for them, but also serves as a catalyst for community action toward the resolution of a common and significant problem.

Glossary

▼

Adjuvant: A substance added to a vaccine formulation that strengthens the immune response to a vaccine antigen.

Antibody: A soluble protein molecule produced and secreted by B cells in response to an antigen which is capable of binding to that specific antigen. Antibodies are induced by vaccine.

Antigen: Any substance that, when introduced into the body, is recognized by the immune system.

Antigenemia: The presence of antigen in the blood.

Antigenic shift: A major, unpredictable change in the surface antigen of a disease-causing organism.

Antigenic variation: A change in the surface antigen of an organism that may help the organism escape destruction by the immune system.

Attenuated: A weakened form of a previously virulent microbe (bacterium or virus) that retains the ability to cause infection without serious symptoms or disease.

Basic research: Studies that are conducted in the laboratory to develop a knowledge base that can be applied in a specific clinical setting.

Blind study: A single-blind study is a clinical trial in which the participant does not know whether s/he is receiving the experimental or the control substance. In a double-blind study, neither the participant nor the research team knows.

Biologicals: Preparations used in the diagnosis, prevention, or treatment of disease which are made from living organisms and their products and act on the immune system.

Booster: An additional dose of a vaccine usually given months to years after the initial vaccine for the purpose of enhancing or "boosting" the immune response.

Carcinogenesis: The production or origin of cancer.

Cell-mediated immunity or cellular immunity: That portion of the immune system mediated by the small white blood cells called T cells or T lymphocytes.

Challenge: In vaccine research, the deliberate introduction of virus or bacteria into previously vaccinated persons or animals (and often controls as well) in order to test the effectiveness of a vaccine. Ideally, the ability of the vaccine to provide protection would be demonstrated by challenge experiments in animals before large-scale human trials were undertaken.

Chimeric virus: A virus composed of a vector into which genes from another virus have been inserted; e.g., vaccinia virus expressing gp160.

Clinical research: Research studies which involve actual observation or treatment of persons. This includes studies which evaluate the action of a new drug, a new vaccine, or other treatment in patients.

Clinical trial: Clinical research on drugs, vaccines, or other interventions which is generally divided into successive phases. The research plan for the study is strict and follows scientific rules. In the case of vaccines, clinical trials must demonstrate the safety and efficacy of a vaccine. Phase I and II trials measure safety and immunogenicity. Phase III trials (which are usually randomized, controlled, and blind) measure safety and efficacy. Phase IV trials involve continued post-marketing surveillance for safety and efficacy.

Clone: (1) A group of genetically identical cells or organisms which all came from a single common ancestor. (2) To reproduce multiple identical copies.

Controlled clinical trial: A study in which researchers give an experimental drug or vaccine to one group of people (the treatment group) while they give another product, or no drug or vaccine, to a second group of similar people (the control group). The results of the two groups are then compared.

Cross-reactivity: When the immune system mistakes one compound for another of similar chemical composition and reacts to it.

Culture: The process of cultivating microorganisms or cells in a special solution that encourages growth.

Cytopathic: Refers to the ability of HIV-1 to cause destruction of the cells that it infects.

Cytotoxic T cells: A subset of T lymphocytes that carry the T8 marker and can kill body cells infected by virus or transformed by cancer.

DNA (deoxyribonucleic acid): A nucleic acid that is found in the cell nucleus of all living cells and is the carrier of genetic information.

Double-blind study: A type of study in which neither the participant nor the research staff knows which treatment the participant is getting. It may be the experimental drug or vaccine, a "control," or a placebo.

Effectiveness: In vaccine research, the measure of a vaccine's ability to protect against disease under "real world" conditions. This is different from **efficacy**, which is the measure of the degree of protectiveness provided by a vaccine under the conditions of a controlled clinical trial.

Efficacy: The effectiveness of a drug, vaccine, or other treatment in clinical conditions.

Endemic: Said of a disease which is common to a particular geographic area.

Epidemic: Said of an infectious disease that affects a large number of people at the same time within a particular population or geographic area.

Epidemiology: The study of the relationships between factors that determine the frequency and distribution of diseases in human populations.

Epitope: A unique shape or marker carried on an antigen's surface, which triggers a corresponding immune response.

Equipoise: A concept describing the ethical position which justifies the conduct of a randomized clinical trial. Randomization is ethical if equipoise (or clinical equipoise) exists, i.e., if the investigator or the expert scientific community is genuinely uncertain as to the comparative merits of the alternatives to be tested. (In other words, it is ethical to randomize participants of a clinical trial to Vaccine A or Vaccine B if it is not yet known or proven that Vaccine A is better than or less toxic than B.)

Gene: The basic unit of genetic material (DNA) that carries the directions a cell uses to perform a specific function, such as making a given protein.

Genetically altered or manipulated: Said of an organism or cell in which the genes have been altered, deleted, or in some way manipulated in order to modify function.

Genome: All of the genetic material in an organism, e.g., a virus.

Herd immunity: The phenomenon whereby the risk of transmission of an infectious disease to an unimmunized person is reduced because a certain number of people within a group are effectively immunized (the immunes protect the susceptibles). This is an important goal of immunization.

Heterologous antigens: Antigens that vary in structure and therefore may require a different immune response.

Homologous antigens: Antigens that have the same structure and are subject to a specific immune response.

Humoral immunity: That portion of the immune system mediated by specific antibodies present in the blood serum and tissue fluids of the body.

Hybrid virus: A virus created by inserting novel viral genes into a viral vector. See also **Chimeric virus** and **Vector**.

Hypervariable: A region of considerable heterogeneity or variability. The viral envelope of HIV is described as hypervariable.

Immune response: The reactions of the immune system to foreign substances, with the goal of protecting the body from infection with invading microbes, or from other disease.

Immune serum globulin: A preparation of immunoglobulins that is used for treatment or prevention.

Immunity: The overall capability of an individual to resist or overcome an infection.

Immunization: A preparation of a modified form of a disease-causing infectious agent given in order to induce an immune response which will protect the person from getting the disease.

Immunoassay: The use of antibodies to identify and quantify substances.

Immunocompetent: Capable of developing an adequate and appropriate immune response.

Immunocompromised: Incapable of developing an adequate or appropriate immune response.

Immunogenicity: The capacity to induce an immune response.

Immunoglobulins: A family of large protein molecules which function as antibodies.

Immunologic memory: The ability of immune components to "remember" an antigen to which they have been sensitized. A stronger and more rapid immune response will occur upon reexposure.

Inactivated: Refers to the use of chemicals, irradiation, or other means to make an antigen noninfectious while retaining its ability to induce an immune response.

Incidence: The rate of occurrence of a disease within a population.

Incubation period: The time period between exposure to an infection and the development of symptoms.

Infectivity: The capacity to cause infection.

Inoculation: Injection of microorganisms, serum, toxin, or immunization.

Institutional review board (IRB): Mandated by law, a group composed of clinicians, scientists, clergy, and others that exists to provide an objective and independent review of any research plan involving human subjects. Its purpose is to ensure that the rights and welfare of the human subjects will be protected and that the proposed research is scientifically and ethically sound.

Intracellular virus: Virus inside cells and therefore not accessible to antibody or humoral immune responses.

In vitro: Conducted in a test tube or in the laboratory.

In vivo: Conducted in the living body.

Latency period: A period of relative inactivity or hidden activity of the virus.

Lentivirus: A type of virus with a "slow" but persistent rate of replication and in which the onset of disease is delayed.

Microbes: Minute living organisms, including bacteria, viruses, fungi, and protozoa. Also referred to as microorganisms.

Molecular biology: A branch of biology which studies the molecules and molecular constituents of biological systems.

Monoclonal antibody: Antibodies produced by a single cell or its identical progeny, specific for a given antigen. As a tool for binding to specific protein molecules, monoclonal antibodies are invaluable in research, medicine, and industry.

Monoclonal anti-idiotypic antibody: Custom-made molecules that are mirror images of disease-causing antigens.

Mucosal immunity: Defense against infectious organisms provided by immune cells and products (e.g., antibody) found in the mucous membranes (e.g., lining the genital tract or the mouth).

Neutralizing antibody: Antibody with the capacity to inactivate virus directly. Considered to be a biologically significant measure of protection.

Nontransforming: Not associated with cancerous proliferation. HIV-1, unlike other human retroviruses, is nontransforming.

Opportunistic infection: An infection in an immunocompromised person caused by an organism that does not usually cause disease in persons with healthy immune systems.

Parenteral: Taken into the body through any route other than the gastrointestinal tract (e.g., via injection).

Pathogen: Disease-producing organism.

Pathogenesis: The development and origin of disease.

Pathogenicity: The ability to produce disease.

PCR (polymerase chain reaction): A laboratory test used to detect the presence of HIV-1 RNA or DNA in the circulating blood.

Placebo: In placebo-controlled clinical trials, a substance given to the control group that contains no active drug or biological. The placebo is usually designed to look like and be administered like the active product.

Plasmid: A ring of DNA often taken from bacteria into which a novel gene is inserted in the process of making recombinant DNA.

Polyvalent: Refers to a vaccine produced from cultures of a number of strains of the same species.

Preclinical evaluation: In clinical research, the preliminary work, including in vitro and animal studies, which must be completed before an application for an Investigational New Drug (IND) is filed with the Food and Drug Administration.

Provirus: A name for the viral DNA which is integrated into the host cell genome.

Randomized clinical trial: A study in which each person is assigned by chance (randomly) to the treatment group or the control group.

Reactivity: The capacity of vaccines to cause adverse reactions in the host.

Recombinant DNA: The product of genetic engineering in which simple organisms such as bacteria, yeast, or mammalian cells in culture can be induced to manufacture quantities of recombinant proteins. The gene for the desired protein is spliced into a plasmid which is then reinserted into the organism from which it came. The recombined DNA directs the organism to produce large quantities of the protein.

Reservoir: In infectious diseases, a source of supply of an infectious agent; e.g., man, animals, plants, or organic matter which allows the infectious agent to live.

Retrovirus: A family of RNA viruses, capable of reverse transcription to DNA, which is then persistently integrated into the host cell genome. HIV is a human retrovirus.

RNA (ribonucleic acid): A nucleic acid found primarily in the cytoplasm of cells. An important function of RNA is to direct the synthesis of proteins.

Seroconvert: To change from a negative to a positive reaction to serological tests, which shows that antibodies have developed.

Serology: The scientific study of blood serum, especially to measure the presence and quantity of specific antibodies.

Seropositive: Producing a positive reaction to serological tests, showing specific antibodies in the blood.

Subunit vaccine: A vaccine that uses one or more components of an infectious agent, rather than the whole, to stimulate an immune response.

Surface antigen: An antigen located on the outer cover of a microorganism, usually unique to that organism. Each different strain of the microorganism will exhibit some different surface antigens.

Surrogate marker: An indicator of changes in clinical disease. Because the length of time it takes HIV-infected persons to develop symptoms is rather long and variable, and presenting symptoms are quite diverse, there continues to be an intensive search for reliable surrogate markers of disease progression or of response to therapies.

Susceptibility: Lack of immunity to an infectious disease.

Synthetic peptide: A vaccine composed of a short chain of amino acids (protein building blocks) prepared in the laboratory (rather than from natural products) made to duplicate the immunogenic proteins of the virus.

T cells: Lymphocytes associated with cell-mediated immunity. T indicates their origin and maturation in the thymus gland.

Teratogenic: Capable of producing a congenital malformation in a fetus.

Therapeutic vaccine: A type of vaccine used to treat a patient after infection, rather than to prevent the infection. The goal is to enhance the patient's immune response.

Toxicity: The degree to which a drug or biological is poisonous or harmful to the host.

Toxins: Substances produced by plants and bacteria that are normally very damaging or poisonous to mammalian cells but usually are immunogenic.

Toxoids: Toxins that have been made nontoxic but which retain their immunogenicity.

Vaccine: A preparation of a modified form of a disease-causing infectious agent given in order to induce an immune response which will protect the person from getting the infectious disease.

Vaccinia-naive: Never having been exposed to vaccinia; this would include all people who never received a smallpox vaccine.

Variolation: Inoculating a patient with pustular material from a smallpox lesion to produce immunity to smallpox.

Vector: A live attenuated vector is a virus or bacterium used to carry selected genes from another infectious agent (e.g., HIV). When administered to an individual, the desired antigenic proteins are produced and elicit an immune response.

Viability: The ability to live, grow, and develop.

Viral antigens: The accessible proteins (epitopes) of a virus to which an immune response occurs.

Viremia: Presence of virus in the blood.

Virulence: Relative power and degree of pathogenicity possessed by organisms to produce disease.

Wild-type virus: Virulent form of a virus.

Notes

▼

1. Of these it is estimated that 6 million are men, 1 million are women; 75 percent of infections were acquired through sexual intercourse, most of which (ratio of 4:1) was heterosexual (Mann).

2. It is worth noting, however, that many who are at risk for HIV infection may not be in a position to make fully autonomous decisions. For example, it is often said that young sexually active women in some developing countries are virtually powerless to insist on "safer sex" or to abstain from sexual activity. Because of cultural norms and power structures, these decisions are made by men, and the ability of these young women to voluntarily avoid risky behavior is therefore compromised.

3. Dr. Rod Hoff of the Vaccine Branch, Division of AIDS, NIAID, estimates the cost of each efficacy trial of an HIV vaccine trial to be approximately $35 million (personal communication, June 1993).

4. Protection from HIV has been demonstrated in a limited number of chimpanzees under ideal conditions, and from SIV in a limited number of monkeys. Whether extrapolation is possible from these studies to protection of humans from various viral strains under field conditions remains to be seen.

5. The Vaccine Branch of the Division of AIDS calculates that more people would be protected (approximately 23,000 according to their model) if a 60 percent effective vaccine were used starting in 1998, instead of waiting until 2001 for a 90 percent effective vaccine (Abstract #POC4505, VIII International Conference on AIDS). Although impressive, this model is somewhat misleading because it is calculated based on almost 100 percent coverage immediately (which is most unlikely), and on a vaccine's ability to prevent infection (which is at least questionable if not unlikely); and it also suggests that proceeding earlier with efficacy trials is justified because a 60 percent effective vaccine may become available sooner. The reality is that whether a vaccine is 60 percent or 90 percent effective will be determined only by doing the trial, and only very limited data available to date give any indication of efficacy.

6. In some cases this is seen as desirable (e.g., poliomyelitis), and in other cases as undesirable (e.g., rubella).

7. For example, as described in chapter 4, a live attenuated *nef*-deleted SIV vaccine has provided protection against SIV in a few monkeys, and an HIV recombinant vaccine in a vaccinia vector has been shown to be immunogenic in some chimps and human subjects.

8. A corollary to the diminished probability of infection is that the median age for infection is often increased. Delay in infection to old age may in some cases carry its own liabilities, since the severity of "childhood" diseases may increase with the age at which the infection occurs (see, for example, Anderson).

9. The market is comparatively small because of limited repeat sales (most people take a vaccine only once or a limited number of times), an undervaluation of

preventive services, underestimate of perceived risk, and limitations imposed by the delivery of health care services.

10. A whole killed cholera vaccine developed in 1896 and believed to be effective was used around the world for more than seventy years. Controlled field trials conducted in the 1960s and 1970s demonstrated that the vaccine was not very effective and that immunization was neither cost-effective nor as beneficial as oral rehydration therapy in reducing mortality from cholera.

11. For an interesting historical description of the gay rights movement see R. Padgug and G. Oppenheimer, "Riding the Tigers: AIDS and the Gay Community," in E. Fee and D. Fox, eds., *AIDS: The Making of a Chronic Disease* (Berkeley: University of California Press, 1992), pp. 245–278.

12. For a good review of the issues and arguments, see R. Levine, 1986, chapter 8.

13. The model of letting patients choose which arm they want was suggested by Robert Veatch in Veatch, 1983, and later described in his book *The Patient as Partner* (1987).

14. See Arno and Feiden, chapter 14, for a good discussion of the pros and cons of parallel track.

15. As printed in *Law, Medicine, and Health Care* 19, nos. 3–4 (1991): 247–258.

16. Only a few authors have written about the differences between vaccine research and drug research, including: Bjune and Gedde-Dahl; Dull and Bryan; Ladimer; Mariner, 1990.

17. Although by definition this is not the primary intent of research (even therapeutic), it often occurs. See also the discussion in chapter 2 regarding HIV-infected persons demanding to participate in clinical drug trials because of a perception of personal benefit, and sometimes because of lack of access to treatment or care otherwise.

18. As Smith and Morrow argue, the assessment and balance of potential benefits and harms may differ depending on the risk of disease and mortality in the community: "A higher level of vaccine-related adverse effects might be acceptable in a trial of a vaccine against a disease that was responsible for many deaths in a community than would be acceptable in a study in a community in which the disease was of smaller public health significance" (p. 81). As discussed in chapter 1, perception of the balance between risks and benefits of a vaccine also changes over time as disease incidence declines (e.g., pertussis).

19. I will avoid the complexities of the debate about personhood as distinguished from human beings or sentient beings. Whatever constitutes personhood, a person or human being is deserving of respect for more than just his/her capacity to be autonomous.

20. Also included under descriptions of the principle of respect for persons is the conviction that persons with diminished autonomy should be protected. I will return to this below.

21. The idea of supplementing but not supplanting liberal values with communitarian values was inspired by an essay by Gutmann (1992).

22. As stated above, social beneficence is also limited by the nonconsequentialist principles of justice and respect for autonomy.

23. Examples:

It is difficult to see how the interests of the individual conflict with the interests of society, except, of course, if the society is not his own. Since the case for the needs of a society are often strong, the rights of the experimental subject and the ethics of the experiment must closely correlate within that society. (Ajayi, p. 61)

Whereas in Western terms selfhood emphasizes the individual, in certain African societies it cannot be extricated from a dynamic system of social relationships, both of kinship and of community as defined by the village. (Barry, p. 1083)

[In] some parts of Latin America and the Caribbean, however, the relationship of the subject with society is not viewed in the same way. Rather, some communities . . . think of each person as a participant in the common efforts of the collective whole. Hence, the life of each person assumes meaning in relation to his role in the community. Accordingly, he is expected to participate in projects that are of interest to the community, putting forward his best effort . . . it is difficult to imagine how the interests of the subject can conflict with those of his community. Since the needs of his community are generally pressing and affect all its members, the rights of the research subject and the ethics of the project must be viewed in the context of the goals that this society has for itself. (LaVertu and Linares, p. 474)

24. Interestingly, Ladimer argues that vaccine research should be considered "clinical" because it is for the direct benefit of the community: "Among the types of medical research considered essentially diagnostic or therapeutic for a patient may be included research directed to the collective benefit of the community, comprised of individuals whose current or future condition will be directly aided through participation as a member of a subject or control group" (p. 113).

25. An interesting model which suggests a way to do this is presented by Hermerén, pp. 359–379.

26. "It is the experience of epidemiologists in many countries that, to an increasing extent, ethical controversies affect and even obstruct public-health work and epidemiological research" (Westrin et al., p. 193).

27. Although, as previously recognized, the degree of voluntariness is influenced by many things.

28. For example, even in the 1993 CIOMS guidelines, which reaffirm the ethical obligation to obtain individualized informed consent (Guideline #1), it is recognized that in some cultures a woman's right to self-determination is not acknowledged, and formal consent may have to be obtained from a man! (p. 34).

29. The successful protection of a few monkeys from SIV challenge after administration of a *nef*-deleted attenuated live virus vaccine, first reported in December 1992 (Muthiah et al.), has led some to reopen the question of live attenuated vaccines for human use. To date (April 1994) no live attenuated vaccine candidate has been prepared for human clinical trials.

30. In 1992, a macaque subspecies (pigtail or Nemestrina) was successfully infected with HIV-1 (FCCSET; Karzon, Bolognesi, and Koff; Schultz and Hu). It remains to be seen if this model will be useful for HIV, because attempts to duplicate the *in vivo* results have met with mixed success. Some studies have shown waning viral replication over the course of a few months, and it is unknown whether disease will occur in these monkeys (Schultz and Hu; FCCSET).

31. The Public Health Service Coolfont Conference recommended a $10,000 lifetime care dowry for each chimpanzee that is experimentally infected with HIV (*Public Health Reports* 101 [1986]: 341–348).

32. The logical extension of this argument is that it is cheaper, easier, and more direct to challenge infected humans with virus than to wait for them to be exposed to natural virus.

33. HIV-2, another human retrovirus with properties similar to those of HIV-1, has common pathogenic potential but only 50 to 60 percent genetic homology with HIV-1. The envelope antigens of HIV-2 are distinct from those of HIV-1 (Katzenstein, Quinnan, and Sawyer); therefore, a vaccine candidate employing HIV-1 envelope antigens would not protect against HIV-2.

34. In some Phase I vaccine studies, seronegative homosexual men were enrolled who promised to abstain from sex or practice safe sex for a period of months before and after receiving the experimental vaccine.

35. The Johns Hopkins Study (one of the five sites) is recruiting six different groups: heterosexual teenagers and young adults (age 16–28) attending an STD clinic

or practicing high-risk sexual behavior; homosexually active men practicing high-risk behavior; homosexually active men practicing low-risk behavior; intravenous drug users active within the past three years; heterosexual partners of HIV seropositive individuals; and adult women and heterosexual men practicing lower-risk sexual behavior (Johns Hopkins University Information Office).

36. The U.S. Congress (1992) allocated $20 million to the Department of Defense to conduct an efficacy trial of MicroGeneSys's gp160 vaccine as therapy in HIV-infected persons. Despite little scientific evidence to support the selective pursuit of gp160 or to support moving any therapeutic vaccine into Phase III trials, Congress passed the legislation. The NIH and FDA convened an expert panel to review the data and address the issue of therapeutic vaccine trials. They recommended a jointly sponsored multicandidate efficacy trial. After many months of debate and the transfer of money back and forth between the Defense Department and NIH, the money was ultimately used by the DOD for basic science and early clinical studies of vaccines in general. This is a perfect example of science misguided by politics.

37. See, for example, Schooley, 1988, and Esparza et al., 1991.

38. Optimal Guidelines: The vaccine candidate should (1) protect animals in challenge studies from HIV infection/disease induced by cell-associated as well as cell-free virus; (2) protect against a broad spectrum of heterologous isolates; (3) protect against intravenous and mucosal challenge; (4) induce long-lasting immunity so that protection occurs if virus is administered months to years after immunization; (5) demonstrate immunological or genetic similarity to HIV isolates from proposed efficacy trial site; and (6) demonstrate induction of correlates of immunity in Phase I clinical trials.

39. In consideration of the current state of HIV vaccine research, core guidelines were established to facilitate the decision-making process for entry of a candidate vaccine into efficacy trials. Safety in Phase I trials plus at least two of the three core guidelines are recommended: (1) demonstrated efficacy in HIV-infected chimps or SIV-infected monkeys; (2) elicited neutralizing antibody which is long-lasting and broadly reactive against heterologous isolates in Phase I trials, strengthened by similar induction of long-term and broadly reactive cellular immunity; (3) demonstrated immunological or genetic similarity to HIV isolates from proposed efficacy trial sites (Final Report of the Ad Hoc HIV Vaccine Advisory Panel, July 1991).

40. At the June 1993 meeting of the Working Group, a session on the ethical and social issues was part of the agenda for the first time. Most of the members agreed that the ethical and social obstacles were enormous and should be dealt with before the initiation of an efficacy trial. The AIDS Action Foundation in collaboration with the NIH Office of AIDS Research held a meeting on social, ethical, and political considerations for domestic HIV vaccine efficacy trials in May 1994.

41. Of interest is an article (David Brown, *Washington Post*, June 10, 1993, p. A13) reporting on presentations from the 9th International AIDS Conference: "Large-scale studies of vaccines designed to prevent infection with the AIDS virus may begin as soon as early 1995—but they may turn out to be more educational to scientists than beneficial to subjects. . . . Even the best designed vaccines of the near future will almost certainly function chiefly as research probes [to determine what confers protection] even if they also happen to protect some people from infection." Dr. B. Haynes writes, "Core criteria . . . may be used to justify entry of an experimental immunogen into a phase III efficacy trial to *answer scientific and clinical questions necessary to direct research and future immunogen design*" (p. 1283; my emphasis).

42. In the U.S., that determination will be made by the Center for Biologics Evaluation and Research of the FDA.

43. Important studies include looking at immune responses in uninfected newborns of infected mothers, persons who remain uninfected despite sexual encounters (sometimes repeated) with infected partners, and HIV-infected long-term survivors,

as well as following over a long period of time some participants of Phase I vaccine studies and of therapeutic vaccine trials.

44. Both individual scientists and companies involved in the development of any vaccine candidate are likely to be biased in their assessment of it. "Because of the potentially great profits likely to accrue to developer and manufacturer of a successful vaccine, the possibility of bias in the enthusiasm of companies for their own product exists despite the best intentions of the companies. Every effort must be made to assure that decisions regarding vaccine selection and interpretation of data are done objectively. Studies comparing vaccines from different manufacturers should be insisted upon, despite the frequent resistance of manufacturers to such studies" (Hoke, p. S163).

45. These four sites were selected from fourteen developing countries visited by a WHO/GPA team in 1991. Selection was based on the epidemiology of HIV, existing clinical and laboratory infrastructure, logistical and operational aspects, community support, and political commitment (Esparza). In October 1994, a WHO panel decided to proceed with efficacy testing of two gp120 subunit vaccine candidates in one of these developing countries. A U.S. panel had decided in June 1994 not to test these products for efficacy now in the U.S.

46. A third functional goal of vaccination for HIV is prevention of transmission. If a vaccine is capable of reducing viral burden in vaccinated subjects exposed to virus, it should also decrease the ability of that individual to transmit virus to sexual partners or to infants during gestation, birth, or breastfeeding. Although extremely important in terms of benefit to society, this goal will probably be met in conjunction with the others. Many vaccines which protect against disease in the recipient also serve to reduce the chances of transmission to others. Vaccines used for therapeutic purposes in already infected persons may also serve to reduce viral burden and therefore transmission. Measuring infection or disease in the individual, although not without problems, is more straightforward than measuring prevention of transmission, and so is traditionally used as a measure of efficacy.

47. In my discussions with the Vaccine Branch of the Division of AIDS, NIAID, scientists identified six possible outcomes of an HIV vaccine efficacy trial: "sterilizing" immunity, aborted infection, modified infection, modified disease, no effect, and enhancement of disease. A "successful" vaccine would be one that resulted in one or more of the first four options. Therefore, meaningful endpoint measurements which could capture any of these different outcomes are essential.

48. As more complicated vaccines or combination vaccines are used, this problem will also become more complicated.

49. One example might be prisoners who, in addition to the risks associated with participation in any drug protocol, are at risk of violence at the hands of other inmates or guards if they are identified as being HIV-infected because they are participating in a trial of an HIV therapy.

50. In June 1993, a Colombian scientist who created a completely synthetic antimalaria vaccine (which is currently undergoing clinical trials and has some very promising preliminary data) transferred the patent rights to the WHO so that the vaccine could be distributed and used by the "poor people of the world." Instead of making a potential multi-million-dollar deal with a pharmaceutical company, he opted to give it to the WHO and said, "I always wanted the recognition and love of the people, and this is an opportunity to get it" (Interview on National Public Radio, June 7, 1993).

51. Novick provides a very useful discussion of the vulnerability of persons likely to be recruited for HIV studies. "The bottom line is that persons with HIV infection [and also those at risk] often belong to groups that are officially deprived of civil rights, disdained, or disrespected. Others are rendered highly vulnerable to coercion by their illness, poverty, or social status. In addition, their cultural values and concerns are often unknown to investigators. Informed consent negotiations, confidentiality procedures, and fairness are all severely threatened by disrespect" (1989, p. 125).

52. The chief of the Vaccine Trials and Epidemiology Branch of the Division of AIDS, NIAID, calculated a sample size for a hypothetical two-arm placebo-controlled efficacy trial. Assuming 90 percent power to detect 50 percent efficacy, and with a 10 percent annual loss to follow-up and 2 percent annual seroincidence, he estimates needing 6,900 subjects for a two-year trial and 3,700 for a three-year trial. He also points out that testing multiple candidates or planning for stratum-specific analyses (e.g., by transmission, by STD status) would require yet higher samples (S. Vermund, submitted 3/23/93 as part of Proceedings on "Models and Methods of Epidemiologic Research in HIV Infection").

53. The FCCSET Working Group Report (1993) states: "Study designs and data collection forms must be sharply focused on a few key measurements, rather than on all possible outcomes. Similarly, laboratory data generation, collection, and analysis must be kept to a streamlined minimum. Banking specimens for testing at a later date can conserve resources and maintain the focus on the most critical analyses" (p. 61)—which makes it all the more essential that the outcomes and measurements to be evaluated are meaningful, agreed upon, and standardized before efficacy trials begin.

54. Interestingly, the efficacy of the recombinant HBV vaccine was demonstrated in neonates born to chronic carrier mothers. There were several reasons for this decision, including that a placebo group could not be used because of an already efficacious plasma-derived vaccine; the sexual habits of gay men (and therefore risk of HBV) had changed because of a fear of AIDS; and HBV infection had also declined in other groups, such as staff and patients in dialysis, so historical data were unreliable. However, in the case of hepatitis B, 70 to 90 percent of babies born to infected mothers are themselves infected, whereas in HIV more than 70 percent remain uninfected. The use of Zidovudine by pregnant women any time after the first trimester was shown in early 1994 to further reduce the incidence of infection in neonates to approximately 8 percent.

55. This is potentially a very serious problem. Unless and until discrimination against persons who test positive for antibody to HIV is reduced or eliminated, those with vaccine-induced antibody, even though they are not infected, will be vulnerable to discrimination on a number of fronts.

56. Two states, California and Connecticut, have passed legislation which grants some product liability relief to HIV vaccine manufacturers in their states, including during the clinical trials process.

57. The FCCSET report, for example, suggests that prison populations in the U.S. may not represent a good study population because the rates of HIV transmission are relatively low (p. 95).

58. However, CIOMS also points out that research involving prisoners as subjects is permitted in very few countries, and is controversial even in those. HIV vaccine research proposing to involve prisoners as volunteers would first have to be permitted in the host country and approved by the appropriate government authorities before potential prison communities were approached.

59. In many of the Phase I vaccine trials, participants were given official documentation of their participation in the form of cards (with a government seal) or western blot strips. In addition, hot lines were established through which participation could be confirmed with the participant's permission.

60. The Office of Technology Assessment, U.S. Congress, is preparing a report (spring 1994) on the issue of compensation for injury from HIV vaccine trials or the use of HIV vaccine postmarketing.

61. Alvin Novick makes an additional case for compensating those who become infected during participation in the trial. Infection would not be considered vaccine-induced injury, but "we depend on data from those who become infected. If everyone remains uninfected, we learn nothing." Novick argues that these individuals deserve compensation for the "risk of progression to a fatal disease, loss of employment, disqualification for health and life insurance and other social harms" (1988, pp. 47–48). Although few others have suggested this, does infection consti-

tute a "physical injury [suffered] as a result of . . . participation"? There is no historical precedent for compensating those who became infected during participation in a vaccine trial.

62. Melton and colleagues suggest bringing in outside leaders or advocates to ensure that participants' views are heard or even to play devil's advocate at the town meetings; assigning each member of the meeting the role of critical evaluator; and delaying the informed consent of individuals and negotiating individual informed consent in private meetings between investigators and potential participants (Melton et al., pp. 577–578).

References

Abram, M., and Wolf, S. 1984. Public Involvement in Medical Ethics: A Model for Government Action. *New England Journal of Medicine* 310: 627–632.

Ackerman, T. 1990. Protectionism and the New Research Imperative in Pediatric AIDS. *IRB: A Review of Human Subjects Research* 12(5): 1–5.

———. 1992. Balancing Moral Principles in Federal Regulations on Human Research. *IRB: A Review of Human Subjects Research* 14(1): 1–6.

Ad Hoc Working Group for the Development of Standards for Pediatric Immunization Practices. 1993. Standards for Pediatric Immunization Practices. *Journal of the American Medical Association* 269: 1817–1822.

Ada, G.; Blanden, B.; and Milbacher, A. 1992. HIV: To Vaccinate or Not to Vaccinate? *Nature* 359: 572.

Ada, G.; Koff, W.; and Petricciani, J. 1992. The Next Steps in HIV Vaccine Development. *AIDS Research and Human Retroviruses* 8(8): 1317–1319.

Ajayi, O. 1980. Taboos and Clinical Research in West Africa. *Journal of Medical Ethics* 6: 61–63.

Aldovini, A., and Young, R. 1992. HIV-1 Virus Like Particles as a Source of Antigen for AIDS Vaccine. In *Vaccine Research and Development*, ed. W. Koff and H. Six, pp. 43–50. New York: Marcel Dekker, Inc.

Aldovini, A.; Young, R.; and Palker, T. 1991. New AIDS Vaccine Candidates: Antigen Delivery and Design. *AIDS* 5(supp. 2): S151–S158.

Allebeck, P., and Jansson, B. 1990. *Ethics in Medicine: Individual Integrity vs Demands of Society*. New York: Raven Press.

Altman, L. K. 1986. Who Will Volunteer for an AIDS Vaccine? *New York Times*, April 15, C1–C8.

———. 1987. *Who Goes First? The Story of Self-Experimentation in Medicine*. New York: Random House.

Anderson, R. 1992. The Concept of Herd Immunity and the Design of Community-Based Immunization Programs. *Vaccine* 10: 928–935.

Angell, M. 1984. Patients' Preferences in Randomized Clinical Trials. *New England Journal of Medicine* 310(21): 1385–1387.

———. 1992. Editorial Responsibility: Protecting Human Rights by Restructuring Publication of Unethical Research. In *The Nazi Doctors and the Nuremberg Code: Human Rights in Human Experimentation*, ed. G. Annas and M. Grodin, pp. 276–285. New York: Oxford University Press.

Annas, G. 1990. Faith (Healing), Hope, and Charity at the FDA: The Politics of AIDS Drug Trials. In *AIDS and the Health Care System*, ed. L. Gostin, pp. 183–196. New Haven: Yale University Press.

———. 1992. The Nuremberg Code in U.S. Courts: Ethics vs. Expediency. In *The Nazi Doctors and the Nuremberg Code: Human Rights in Human Experi-*

mentation, ed. G. Annas and M. Grodin, pp. 201–222. New York: Oxford University Press.

Annas, G., and Grodin, M. 1992. Where Do We Go from Here? In *The Nazi Doctors and the Nuremberg Code: Human Rights in Human Experimentation*, ed. G. Annas and M. Grodin, pp. 307–314. New York: Oxford University Press.

Applebaum, P.; Roth, L.; Lidz, C.; Beeson, P.; and Winslade, W. 1987. False Hopes and Best Data: Consent to Research and the Therapeutic Misconception. *Hastings Center Report* 17: 20–24.

Archer, S. 1979. Community. In *Community Health Nursing*, ed. S. Archer and R. Fleshman, pp. 22–54. North Scituate, Mass.: Duxbury Press.

Arno, P., and Feiden, K. 1992. *Against the Odds: The Story of AIDS Drug Development, Politics, and Profits*. New York: Harper-Collins Publishers, Inc.

Avineri, S., and deShalit, A. 1992. *Communitarianism and Individualism*. New York: Oxford University Press.

Baker, C., and Brennan, J. 1984. Keeping Health Care Workers Healthy: Legal Aspects of Hepatitis B Immunization Program. *New England Journal of Medicine* 311(10): 684–688.

Banatvala, J., and Best, J. 1989. Rubella Vaccines. In *Recent Developments in Prophylactic Immunizations*, ed. A. Zuckerman, pp. 155–180. Dordrecht: Kluwer Publishers.

Bankhead, C. 1984. Patients Can Become Victims in Some Clinical Trials. *Medical World News* 25(4): 68–69.

Barber, B. 1976. The Ethics of Experimentation with Human Subjects. *Scientific American* 234(2): 25–31.

Barber, B.; Lally, J.; Makarustika, J.; and Sullivan, D. 1973. *Research on Human Subjects: Problems in Social Control in Medical Experimentation*. New York: Russell Sage Foundation.

Barnes, D. 1986. Will an AIDS Vaccine Bankrupt the Company That Makes It? *Science* 233: 1035.

Barrick, B.; Berkebile, C.; Cuda, S.; Govoni, L.; Grady, C.; Hahn, B.; Rosenthal, Y.; Sears, N.; and Megill, M. 1988. Motivations of Persons Volunteering for an AIDS Vaccine Trial. *IV International Conference on AIDS* #6575 (Abstract).

Barry, M. 1988. Ethical Considerations of Human Investigation in Developing Countries: The AIDS Dilemma. *New England Journal of Medicine* 319: 1083–1085.

Baum, M. 1982. The Ethics of Clinical Trials and Informed Consent. *Experientia Supp.* 4: 300–308.

———. 1986. Do We Need Informed Consent? *Lancet* 2(8512): 911–912.

Baum, M.; Zekaa, K.; and Houghton, J. 1989. Ethics of Clinical Research: Lessons for the Future. *British Medical Journal* 299(6693): 251–253.

Bay, C. 1978. From Contract to Community: Thoughts on Liberalism and Post-industrial Society. In *From Contract to Community*, ed. F. Dallmayr, pp. 29–45. New York: Marcel Dekker.

Bayer, R. 1991. *Private Acts, Social Consequences*. New Brunswick, N.J.: Rutgers University Press.

Bayer, R., and Gostin, L. 1990. Legal and Ethical Issues Related to AIDS. In *Bioethics Issues and Perspectives*, ed. S. Connor and H. Fuenzalida-Puelma, pp. 94–115. Washington, D.C.: PAHO.

Beale, A. 1988. Vaccine Development Reconsidered. *Vaccine* 6(2): 138–140.

Beauchamp, T., and Childress, J. 1989. *Principles of Biomedical Ethics*. 3rd ed. New York: Oxford University Press.

Beecher, H. K. 1966. Ethics and Clinical Research. *New England Journal of Medicine* 274: 1354–1360.

———. 1970a. The Subject. In *Research and the Individual: Human Studies*, pp. 33–78. Boston: Little, Brown and Company.

———. 1970b. Science in Research Trials: Moral, Ethical, and Religious Issues. In

Research and the Individual: Human Studies, pp. 185–212. Boston: Little Brown and Company.

Begg, N., and Miller, E. 1990. Role of Epidemiology in Vaccine Policy. *Vaccine* 8: 180–189.

Bellah, R.; Madsen, R.; Sullivan, W.; Swidler, A.; and Tipton, S. 1985. *Habits of the Heart: Individualism and Commitment in American Life*. Berkeley: University of California Press.

Benenson, A. 1990. *Control of Communicable Diseases in Man*. 15th ed. Washington, D.C.: APHA.

Berger, E. 1989. The Expression of Health Risk Influence. *Archives of Internal Medicine* 149: 1507–1508.

Bergkamp, C. 1989. The Rise of Research Ethics Committees in Western Europe. *Bioethics* 3(2): 122–134.

Berman, P.; Gregory, T.; Riddle, L.; et al. 1990. Protection of Chimpanzees from Infection by HIV-1 Vaccination with Recombinant Glycoprotein 120 but Not gp160. *Nature* 345: 622–625.

Bernier, R. 1990. Outstanding Issues in the Clinical Evaluation of New Acellular Pertussis Vaccines. In *Proceedings of the Sixth International Symposium on Pertussis*, ed. C. Manclark, pp. 311–314. Bethesda: DHHS, USPHS.

Bjune, G., and Arnesen, O. 1992. Problems Related to Consent from Young Teenagers Participating in Efficacy Testing of a New Vaccine. *IRB: A Review of Human Subjects Research* 14(5): 6–9.

Bjune, G., and Gedde-Dahl, T. 1993. Some Problems Related to Risk-Benefit Assessments in Clinical Trials of New Vaccines. *IRB: A Review of Human Subjects Research* 15(1): 1–5.

Black, F., and Sheridan, S. 1960. Studies of Attenuated Measles Virus Vaccine: Administration of Vaccine by Several Routes. *New England Journal of Medicine* 263: 165–169.

Bloom, B. 1989. Vaccines for the Third World. *Nature* 342: 115–120.

Blum, H. 1974. Implementation: Conversion of Plans into Policy and Operations. In *Planning for Health: Development and Application of Social Change Theory*, ed. H. Blum, pp. 476–541. New York: Human Sciences Press.

Bracken, M. 1987. Clinical Trials and the Acceptance of Uncertainty. *British Medical Journal* 294(6580): 1111–1112.

Bradac, J., and Ho, D. 1992. Summary of Antigenic Variation Working Group. *AIDS Research and Human Retroviruses* 8(8): 1419–1421.

Brahams, D. 1982. Clinical Trials and the Consent of the Patient. *The Practitioner* 226: 1829–1830.

Brandt, A. 1978a. Polio: Politics, Publicity, and Duplicity. *International Journal of Health Services* 8(2): 257–270.

———. 1978b. Racism and Research: The Case of the Tuskegee Syphilis Study. *Hastings Center Report* 8(6): 21–29.

———. 1988. AIDS in Historical Perspective: Four Lessons from the History of Sexually Transmitted Diseases. *American Journal of Public Health* 78(4): 367–371.

Brandt, E. 1988. Hard Choices in Public Health. *Public Health Reports* 103: 339–341.

Brett, A., and Grodin, M. 1991. Ethical Aspects of Human Experimentation in Health Services Research. *Journal of the American Medical Association* 265(4): 1854–1857.

Brock, D. 1987. Informed Consent. In *Health Care Ethics*, ed. Van D. DeVeer and T. Regan, pp. 98–126. Philadelphia: Temple University Press.

Broder, S. 1989. Controlled Trial Methodology and Progress in the Treatment of AIDS: A Quid Pro Quo. *Annals of Internal Medicine* 110(6): 417–418.

Brown, P. 1991. AIDS Vaccines: What Chance of a Fair Trial? *New Scientist* 130(1766): 33–37.

Bujoran, G. 1988. Clinical Trials: Patient Issues in the Decision Making Process. *Oncology Nursing Forum* 15(6): 779–783.

Burckhardt, R., and Keinle, G. 1978. Controlled Clinical Trials and Medical Ethics. *Lancet* 2: 8104–8105.

Burnette, W. 1992a. Perspectives in Recent Pertussis Toxoid Development. In *Vaccine Research and Development*, vol. 1, ed. W. Koff and H. Six, pp. 143–171. New York: Marcel Dekker, Inc.

———. 1992b. Vaccine Development: Necessity as the Mother of Invention. *The New Biologist* 4: 269–273.

Butler, J. 1978. Is It Ethical to Conduct Volunteer Studies within the Pharmaceutical Industry? *Lancet* 1: 816–818.

Byar, D. 1977. Sound Advice for Conducting Clinical Trials. *New England Journal of Medicine* 297(10): 553–554.

———. 1990. Design Considerations for AIDS Trials. *New England Journal of Medicine* 323(19): 1343–1348.

Calabresi, G. 1970. Reflections on Medical Experimentation in Humans. In *Experimentation with Human Subjects*, ed. P. Freund, pp. 178–196. New York: George Braziller.

Callahan, D. 1981. Minimalist Ethics. *Hastings Center Report* 11(5): 19–25.

———. 1990. *What Kind of Life? The Limits of Medical Progress.* New York: Simon and Schuster.

Caplan, A. 1984. Is There a Duty to Serve as a Subject in Biomedical Research? *IRB: A Review of Human Subjects Research* 6(5): 1–5.

———. 1992a. The Doctor's Trial and Analogies to the Holocaust in Contemporary Bioethical Debates. In *The Nazi Doctors and the Nuremberg Code: Human Rights in Human Experimentation*, ed. G. Annas and M. Grodin, pp. 258–275. New York: Oxford University Press.

———. 1992b. The Tuskegee Legacy: When Evil Intrudes. *Hastings Center Report* 22: 29–32.

Capron, A. 1983a. Ethics of Phase I Clinical Trials. *Journal of the American Medical Association* 249(7): 882–883.

———. 1983b. Prospects for Research Ethics. In *Research Ethics*, ed. K. Berg and K. Tranoy, pp. 389–397. New York: Alan R. Liss, Inc.

———. 1991. Protection of Research Subjects: Do Special Rules Apply in Epidemiology? *Law, Medicine and Health Care* 19: 184–190.

Cardon, P.; Dammel, W.; and Trumble, R. 1976. Injuries to Research Subjects. *New England Journal of Medicine* 295: 650–654.

Carter, M.; McCarthy, R.; and Wichman, A. 1990. The Moral Task of IRBs. *Bridges* 2(1–2): 63–73.

Carter, S. 1978. Clinical Trials. *Cancer Immunology and Immunotherapy* 3: 215–218.

Cassileth, B.; Zyskes, R.; Sutton-Smith, K.; and March, B. 1980. Informed Consent: Why Are Its Goals Imperfectly Realized? *New England Journal of Medicine* 302(16): 896–900.

Catania, J.; Coates, T.; and Stall, R. 1992. Prevention of AIDS: Related to Risk Factors and Condom Use in the United States. *Science* 258: 1101–1106.

Cates, W., and Hinman, A. 1992. AIDS and Absolutism: The Demand for Perfection in Prevention. *New England Journal of Medicine* 327(7): 492–494.

Challice, J. 1992. AIDS Research: An Interview with Jean-Claude Cherman. *PAAC-NOTES* 4(3): 120–124.

Chalmers, T. 1975. Ethical Aspects of Clinical Trials. *American Journal of Ophthalmology* 79: 753–758.

———. 1981. The Clinical Trial. *Milbank Memorial Fund Quarterly* 59: 325–339.

———. 1990. Ethical Implications of Rejecting Patients for Clinical Trials. *Journal of the American Medical Association* 263(6): 865.

Chalmers, T.; Celano, P.; Sacks, H.; and Smith, H. 1983. Bias in Medication Assignment with Controlled Clinical Trials. *New England Journal of Medicine* 309(22): 1358–1361.

Chalmers, T.; Van de Noort, S.; and Lackshen, T. 1983. Summary of Workshop on Role of Third Party Payers in Clinical Trials of New Agents. *New England Journal of Medicine* 309(21): 1334–1336.

Chang, T.; Desrosiers, S.; and Weinstein, L. 1970. Clinical and Serological Studies of an Outbreak of Rubella in a Vaccinated Population. *New England Journal of Medicine* 283: 246–248.

Chanock, R. 1990. Control of Pediatric Viral Diseases: Past Successes and Future Prospects. *Pediatric Research* 27(supp. 6): S39–S43.

Chanock, R.; Parrot, R.; Connors, M.; Collins, P.; and Murphy, B. 1992. Serious Respiratory Tract Disease Caused by Respiratory Syncytial Virus: Prospects for Improved Therapy and Effective Immunization. *Pediatrics* 90: 137–142.

Check, W. 1984. How to Remedy Possible Harm to a Few Persons from Vaccines That Could Benefit Entire Society? *Journal of the American Medical Association* 252(21): 2942–2946.

Cherry, J.; McIntosh, K.; Connor, J.; Benenson, A.; Alling, D.; Rolfe, U.; Todd, W.; Schauberger, J.; and Mattheis, M. 1977. Primary Percutaneous Smallpox Vaccination. *Journal of Infectious Diseases* 135: 145–154.

Christakis, N. 1988. The Ethical Design of an AIDS Vaccine Trial in Africa. *Hastings Center Report* 18(3): 31–37.

———. 1992. Ethics Are Local: Engaging Cross-Cultural Variation in the Ethics for Clinical Research. *Social Science and Medicine* 35: 1079–1091.

Christakis, N., and Panner, M. 1991. Existing International Guidelines for Health Services Research: Some Open Questions. *Law, Medicine, and Health Care* 19(3–4): 214–221.

CIOMS. See *Council for International Organizations of Medical Sciences*

Clemens, J.; Harris, J.; and Khan, M. 1986. Field Trial of Oral Cholera Vaccine in Bangladesh. *Lancet* 2: 124–126.

Clemens, J.; VanLoon, F.; Rao, M.; Sack, D.; Ahmed, F.; Chakraborty, J.; Khan, M.; Yumus, M.; Harris, J.; Svennerholm, A.; and Holmgren, J. 1992. Nonparticipation as a Determinant of Adverse Health Outcomes in a Field Trial of Oral Cholera Vaccines. *American Journal of Epidemiology* 135: 865–874.

Cockburn, W. 1977. Disease Control and Prevention in the 20th Century: The Role of Immunization. *Bulletin of the WHO* 55(supp. 2): 3–18.

Cohen, C. 1977. When May Research Be Stopped? *New England Journal of Medicine* 296: 1203–1210.

Cohen, J. 1991. AIDS Vaccine Trials: Bumpy Road Ahead. *Science* 251: 1312–1313.

———. 1992a. AIDS Vaccines: Is Older Better? *Science* 258: 1880–1881.

———. 1992b. Pediatric AIDS Vaccine Trials Set. *Science* 258: 1568–1570.

———. 1993. AIDS Research: The Mood Is Uncertain. *Science* 260: 1254–1261.

Cohen, S. 1977. Development of Drug Prescriptions for Children. *Federalism Proceedings* 36(10): 2356–2358.

Coles, P., and Anderson, C. 1991. Inquiry Launched into Ethical Procedures. *Nature* 350(6315): 179.

Cooper, E. 1988. Controlled Clinical Trials of AIDS Drugs: The Best Hope. *Journal of the American Medical Association* 261(16): 2445.

Council for International Organizations of Medical Sciences. 1982. *Proposed International Guidelines for Biomedical Research Involving Human Subjects.* Geneva: CIOMS/WHO.

———. 1991. *International Guidelines for Review of Epidemiological Studies.* Geneva: CIOMS/WHO.

———. 1992. *Draft International Ethical Guidelines for Biomedical Research Involving Human Subjects.* Geneva: CIOMS/WHO.

————. 1993. *International Ethical Guidelines for Biomedical Research Involving Human Subjects.* Geneva: CIOMS/WHO.

Cournand, A. 1977. The Code of the Scientist and Its Relationship to Ethics. *Science* 198: 699–705.

Crane, D. 1977. Sociological Perspectives on Biologicals Research in Human Populations. *Bulletin of the WHO* 55(supp. 2): 91–100.

Crooks, G. 1985. Health Policy Making in America: The Process of Building Consensus. *CIOMS XVIIIth Roundtable: Health Policy, Ethics and Human Values* 22–30.

Culliton, B. 1977. Science, Society and the Press. *New England Journal of Medicine* 296(25): 1450–1453.

————. 1991. AIDS Trials Questioned. *Nature* 350: 263.

Curran, W. 1975. Public Warnings of the Risk in Oral Polio Vaccine. *American Journal of Public Health* 65(5): 501–502.

————. 1977. Influence of the Courts of Law on Biologics Development, Regulation, and Use. *Bulletin of the WHO* 55(supp. 2).

————. 1978. Legal Liability in Clinical Investigations. *New England Journal of Medicine* 298(14): 778–779.

Cutts, F; Zell, E.; and Stat, M. 1992. Monitoring Progress by U.S. Preschool Immunization Goals. *Journal of the American Medical Association* 267(14): 1952–1955.

Dahan, R.; Caulen, C.; and Figea, L. 1986. Does Informed Consent Influence Therapeutic Outcome? *British Medical Journal* 293: 363–364.

Davis, W.; Larson, H.; Simsarian, J.; Parkman, P.; and Meyer, H. 1971. A Study of Rubella Immunity and Resistance to Infection. *Journal of the American Medical Association* 215: 600–608.

Degner, L., and Sloan, J. 1992. Decision Making during Severe Illness: What Role Do Patients Really Want to Play? *Journal of Clinical Epidemiology* 45(9): 941–950.

De Grazia, D. 1992. Moving Forward in Bioethical Theory: Theories, Cases and Specified Principles. *Journal of Medicine and Philosophy* 17: 571–539.

Des Jarlais, D., and Stephenson, B. 1991. History, Ethics, and Politics in AIDS Prevention Research. *American Journal of Public Health* 81(11): 1393–1394.

Detels, R.: Grayston, J.; Kim, K.; Chen, K.; Gale, J.; Beasley, R.; and Gutman, L. 1969. Prevention of Clinical and Subclinical Rubella Infection. *American Journal of Diseases of Children* 118: 295–300.

Deutsch, E. 1985. Controlled Clinical Trials in Drug Research: Starting by Permission vs. Notification. *Medicine and Law* 4: 493–497.

Devine, P. 1991. AIDS and the L-word. *Public Affairs Quarterly* 5(2): 137–147.

Diamond, A., and Lawrence, D. 1983. Guidelines: Clinical Trials—Compensation for Injury. *British Medical Journal* 287: 675–677.

Dickens, B.; Gostin, L.; and Levine, R. 1991. Research on Human Populations: National and International Ethical Guidelines. *Law, Medicine, and Health Care* 19(3–4): 157–161.

Dixon, J. 1990. *Catastrophic Rights: Experimental Drugs and AIDS.* Vancouver: New Star Books.

Dorozynski, A., and Anderson, A. 1991. Deaths in Vaccine Trials Trigger French Inquiry. *Science* 252: 501–502.

Douard, J. 1990. Ethics, AIDS, and Community Reponsibility. *Theoretical Medicine* 11: 213–226.

Dowling, H. 1977. *Fighting Infection: Conquests of the 20th Century.* Cambridge, Mass.: Harvard University Press.

Dubler, N., and Sidel, V. 1990. On Research on HIV Infection and AIDS in Correctional Institutions. *The Milbank Quarterly* 67(2): 171–207.

Dudley, H. 1984. Informed Consent in Surgical Trials. *British Medical Journal* 289(6450): 937–938.

Dull, H., and Bryan, J. 1977. Assuring the Benefits of Immunization in the Future: Research in the Public Interest. *Bulletin of the WHO* 55(supp. 2): 117–126.

Dworkin, G. 1978. Legality of Consent to Nontherapeutic Medical Research in Infants and Young Children. *Archives of Diseases in Childhood* 53: 443–446.

Earrickson, R. 1990. International Behavioral Responses to a Health Hazard: AIDS. *Social Science and Medicine* 31(9): 951–962.

Edgar, H. 1992. The Tuskegee Legacy: Outside the Community. *Hastings Center Report* 22: 32–35.

Edgar, H., and Rothman, D. 1990. New Rules for New Drugs: The Challenge of AIDS to the Regulatory Process. *The Milbank Quarterly* 68(supp. 1): 111–142.

Edwards, K.; Decker, M.; and Graham, B. 1993. Adult Immunizations with Acellular Pertussis Vaccine. *Journal of the American Medical Association* 269(1): 53–56.

Eisenberg, L. 1977. The Social Imperatives of Medical Research. *Science* 198: 1105–1110.

———. 1986. The Genesis of Fear: AIDS and the Public—Response to Science. *Law, Medicine, and Health Care* 14(5–6): 243–249.

Ellenberg, S. 1984. Randomization Designs in Comparative Clinical Trials. *New England Journal of Medicine* 310(21): 1404–1408.

Ellis, R. 1988. New Technologies for Making Vaccines. In *Vaccines*, ed. S. Plotkin and E. Mortimer, pp. 568–575. Philadelphia: W. B. Saunders.

———. 1990. Recombinant-Derived Hepatitis B Vaccine. In *AIDS Vaccine Research and Clinical Trials*, ed. S. Putney and D. Bolognesi, pp. 381–408. New York: Marcel Dekker, Inc.

Emanuel, E. J. 1991. *The Ends of Human Life: Medical Ethics in a Liberal Polity.* Cambridge, Mass.: Harvard University Press.

Enders, J., and Katz, S. 1959. Immunization of Children and Live Attenuated Measles Virus. *American Journal of Diseases of Children* 98: 605–607.

Enel, P.; Charrel, J.; Larher, M. P.; Reviron, D.; Manuel, C.; and San Marco, J. L. 1991. Ethical Problems Raised by Anti-HIV Vaccination. *European Journal of Epidemiology* 7(2): 147–153.

Engelhardt, H. T. 1986. *The Foundations of Bioethics.* New York: Oxford University Press.

———. 1988. Diagnosing Well and Treating Prudently: Randomized Clinical Trials and the Problem of Knowing Truly. In *The Use of Human Beings in Research*, ed. S. F. Spicker, I. Alon, A. de Vries, and H. T. Engelhardt, pp. 123–141. Dordrecht: Kluwer Academic Publishers.

Erhardt, A. 1992. Trends in Sexual Behavior and the HIV Pandemic. *American Journal of Public Health* 82(11): 1459–1461.

Esparza, J. 1993. WHO-GPA Vaccine Endeavors: Progress and Expectations. *AIDS Research and Human Retroviruses* 9(supp. 1): S133–S135.

Esparza, J.; Homsy, J.; Widdus, R.; and Mann, J. 1989. International Testing of Candidate Vaccines for HIV: Scientific, Ethical, Social, and Legal Issues. In *Vaccines for Sexually Transmitted Diseases*, ed. A. Meheus and R. E. Spier, pp. 298–304. London: Butterworths and Co. Ltd.

Esparza, J.; Osmanov, S.; Kallings, L.; and Wigzell, H. 1991. Planning for HIV Vaccine Trials: The WHO Perspective. *AIDS* 5(supp. 2): S159–S163.

Fast, P., and Walker, M. 1993. Human Trials of Experimental AIDS Vaccines. *AIDS* 7(supp. 1): S147–S159.

Fauci, A. 1991. Optimal Immunity to HIV: Natural Infection, Vaccination, or Both? *New England Journal of Medicine* 324(24): 1733–1735.

Fauci, A.; Gallo, R.; Koenig, S.; Salk, J.; and Purcell, R. 1989. Development and Evaluation of a Vaccine for Human Immunodeficiency Virus (HIV) infection. *Annals of Internal Medicine* 110(5): 373–385.

Federal Coordinating Committee on Science, Engineering, and Technology (FCCSET). 1993. *Report of the Working Group on HIV Vaccine Development and International Field Trials*. Washington, D.C.: FCCSET.

Feeley, J., and Gangarosa, E. 1980. Field Trials of Cholera Vaccine. In *Cholera and Related Diarrheas*, ed. O. Ouchterlony and J. Holmgren, pp. 204–210. Basel: Karger.

Fenner, F. 1985. Vaccination: Its Birth, Death, and Resurrection. *Australian Journal of Experimental Biology and Medical Science* 63(pt. 6): 607–622.

Fetter, M.; Feetham, S.; and D'Apolito, K. 1989. Randomized Clinical Trials: Issues for Research. *Nursing Research* 38(2): 117–120.

Fine, P., and Clarkson, J. 1986. Individual vs. Public Problems in the Development of Optimal Vaccination Policies. *American Journal of Epidemiology* 124(6): 1012–1020.

Fineberg, H., and Havson, C. 1992. The Ricochet of Magic Bullets: Summary of the Institute of Medicine Report—Adverse Effects of Pertussis and Rubella Vaccines. *Pediatrics* 89(2): 318–324.

Finkelstein, R. 1984. Cholera. In *Bacterial Vaccines*, ed. R. Germanier, pp. 107–136. New York: New York Academic Press.

Finn, A., and Plotkin, S. 1991. Immunization. In *Harrison's Principles of Internal Medicine*, 12th ed., ed. G. Wilson, E. Braunwald, K. Isselbacher, R. Petersdorf, J. Martin, A. Fauci, and R. Root, pp. 472–478. New York: McGraw Hill.

Fischinger, P. 1989. Progress in Vaccine Development against AIDS. *AIDS Update* 2(4): 1–10.

Fleming, A.; Carballo, M.; and Fitzsimmons, D. 1988. *The Global Impact of AIDS*. New York: Alan Liss, Inc.

Fletcher, J. 1977. Ethical Considerations in Biomedical Research Involving Human Beings. *Bulletin of the WHO* 55(supp. 2): 101–110.

Fletcher, J. C. 1983. The Evolution of the Ethics of Informed Consent. In *Research Ethics*, ed. K. Berg and K. Tranoy, pp. 187–228. New York: Alan Liss, Inc.

Fletcher, R.; Fletcher, S.; and Wagner, E. 1988. *Clinical Epidemiology: The Essentials*. Baltimore: Williams and Wilkins.

Fogel, A.; Handsher, R.; and Bernea, B. 1985. Subclinical Rubella in Pregnancy-Occurrence and Outcome. *Israeli Journal of Medical Science* 21: 133–138.

Forbes, J. 1981. Considerations for a Clinician before Supporting a Clinical Trial. *Australia and New Zealand Journal of Surgery* 51(1): 4–5.

Forrest, B. 1991. Women, HIV, and Mucosal Immunity. *Lancet* 337: 835–836.

———. 1992. Mucosal Approaches to HIV Vaccine Development. *AIDS Research and Human Retroviruses* 8(8): 1523–1525.

Francis, D. 1992. Toward a Comprehensive HIV Prevention Program for the CDC and the Nation. *Journal of the American Medical Association* 268(11): 1444–1447.

Francis, T.; Korns, R.; Voight, R.; Boisen, M.; Hemphill, F.; Napier, J.; and Tolchinsky, E. 1955. An Evaluation of the 1954 Poliomyelitis Vaccine Trials: Summary Report. *American Journal of Public Health* 45(5, pt. 2): 1–63.

Freedman, B. 1987a. Equipoise and the Ethics of Clinical Research. *New England Journal of Medicine* 317(3): 141–145.

———. 1987b. Scientific Value and Validity as Ethical Requirements for Research: A Proposed Explanation. *IRB: A Review of Human Subjects Research* 9(5): 7–10.

———. 1990. Placebo Controlled Trials and the Logic of Clinical Purpose. *IRB: A Review of Human Subjects Research* 12(6): 1–5.

———. 1991. Violating Confidentiality to Warn of a Risk of HIV Infection: Ethical Work in Progress. *Theoretical Medicine* 12: 309–323.

———. 1992. Suspended Judgement: AIDS and the Ethics of Clinical Trials—Learning the Right Lessons. *Controlled Clinical Trials* 13: 1–5.

Freedman, B., and the McGill Boston Research Group. 1989. Nonvalidated Therapies and HIV Disease. *Hastings Center Report* 19(3): 14–20.

Freund, P. 1969. Legal Frameworks for Human Experimentation. In *Experimenta-*

tion with Humans, ed. P. Freund, pp. 105–115. New York: George Braziller.

Fried, C. 1974. *Medical Experimentation: Personal Integrity and Social Policy.* Amsterdam: North-Holland Publishing Co.

Friedman, L., and Howard, J. 1981. Protecting the Scientific Integrity of a Clinical Trial: Some Ethical Dilemmas. *Clinical Pharmacology and Therapeutics* 29(5): 561–569.

Furukawa, T.; Miyata, T.; Kanda, K.; Juno, K.; et al. 1970. Rubella Vaccination during an Epidemic. *Journal of the American Medical Association* 213: 987–990.

Galasso, G.; Mattheis, M.; Cherry, J.; Connor, J.; McIntosh, K.; Benenson, A.; and Alling, D. 1977. Smallpox Vaccination Meeting: Summary. *Journal of Infectious Diseases* 135: 183–186.

Garrett, T.; Baillie, H.; and Garrett, R. 1993. *Health Care Ethics: Principles and Problems.* Englewood Cliffs, N.J.: Prentice Hall, Inc.

Geison, G. 1978. Pasteur's Work on Rabies: Reexamining the Ethical Issues. *Hastings Center Report* 8(2): 26–33.

Gillman, M., and Runyan, D. 1984. Bias in Prescription Assignment in Controlled Clinical Trials. *New England Journal of Medicine* 310(24): 1610–1612.

Glantz, L. 1992. The Influence of the Nuremberg Code on U.S. Statutes and Regulations. In *The Nazi Doctors and the Nuremberg Code: Human Rights in Human Experimentation,* ed. G. Annas and M. Grodin, pp. 183–199. New York: Oxford University Press.

Global Programme on AIDS. 1992. Potential Vaccine Strategies Using HIV Vaccines in Developing Countries. Geneva: WHO/GPA.

Goodman, L., and Goodman, M. 1986. Prevention: How Misuse of a Concept Undercuts Its Worth. *Hastings Center Report* 16: 26–38.

Gordon, R. 1985. The Design and Conduct of Randomized Clinical Trials. *IRB: A Review of Human Subjects Research* 7(1): 1–3, 12.

Gore, S. 1981. Assessing Clinical Trials: First Steps. *British Medical Journal* 282(6276): 1605–1607.

Gostin, L. 1987. Vaccination for AIDS: Legal and Ethical Challenges from the Test Tube, to the Human Subject, through to the Marketplace. *AIDS and Public Policy Journal* 2: 9–16.

———. 1990. *AIDS and the Health Care System.* New Haven: Yale University Press.

———. 1991. Ethical Principles for the Conduct of Human Subjects Research: Population-Based Research and Ethics. *Law, Medicine, and Health Care* 19: 191–201.

———. 1992. The Ethics of Human Subjects Research: WHO/CIOMS Recommend New Guidelines for International Clinical Trials. *PAACNOTES* 4(3): 113–124.

Goudeau, A.; Dubois, F.; and Klein, J. 1988. Vaccine Formulations and Dose Regimen. In *Applied Virology Research: New Vaccines and Chemotherapy Medications,* ed. E. Kusak, R. Marusyk, F. Murphy, and M. VanRegnotel, pp. 195–208. New York: Plenum Medical Books.

Gould, S. 1987. The Terrifying Normalcy of AIDS. *New York Times,* April 19, 33.

Grady, C. 1991. Ethical Issues in Clinical Trials. *Seminars in Oncology Nursing* 7(4): 288–296.

Graham, B.; Belshe, R.; Clements, M.; Dolin, R.; Corey, L.; Wright, P.; Gorse, G.; Midthun, K.; Keefer, M.; Roberts, N.; Schwartz, D.; Agosti, J.; Fernie, B.; Stablein, D.; Montefiori, D.; Lambert, J.; Hu, S.; Esterlitz, J.; Lawrence, D.; Koff, W.; and the AIDS Vaccine Clinical Trials Network. 1992. Vaccination of Vaccinia-Naive Adults with HIV Type 1 gp160 Recombinant Vaccinia Virus in a Blinded, Controlled, Randomized Clinical Trial. *Journal of Infectious Diseases* 166: 244–252.

Graham, L. 1978. Concerns about Science and Attempts to Regulate Inquiry.

Daedalus 107: 1–17.

Grasbeck, R. 1983. The Ultimate Goals of Medical Research. In *Research Ethics*, ed. K. Berg and K. Tranoy, pp. 380–388. New York: Alan Liss, Inc.

Gray, B. 1975. *Human Subjects in Medical Experimentation*. New York: J. Wiley and Sons.

Gray, B.; Cooke, R.; and Tannenbaum, A. 1978. Research Involving Human Subjects. *Science* 201: 1094–1101.

Grayston, J.; Detels, R.; Chen, K.; Gutman, L.; et al. 1969. Field Trial of Live Attenuated Rubella Virus Vaccine during an Epidemic on Taiwan. *Journal of the American Medical Association* 207: 1107–1110.

Grodin, M.; Kaminow, P.; and Sassower, R. 1986. Ethical Issues in AIDS Research. *QRB* 4(1): 347–352.

Grossman, M., and Cohen, S. 1991. Immunization. In *Basic and Clinical Immunology*, 7th ed., ed. D. Stites and A. Terr, pp. 723–741. Norwalk: Lange Medical Book.

Gutmann, A. 1992. Communitarian Critics of Liberalism. In *Communitarianism and Individualism*, ed. S. Avineri and A. deShalit, pp. 120–137. Oxford: Oxford University Press.

Hall, A. 1989. Public Health Trials in West Africa: Logistics and Ethics. *IRB: A Review of Human Subjects Research* 11(5): 8–10.

Hall, S. 1992. Should Public Health Respect Autonomy? *Journal of Medical Ethics* 18: 197–201.

Halstead, S. 1992. Children's Vaccine Initiative. *AIDS Research and Human Retroviruses* 8(8): 1533.

Hamilton, M. 1981. Role of an Ethicist in the Conduct of Clinical Trials in the United States. *Controlled Clinical Trials* 1: 411–420.

Harrington, M. 1992. Constituency Priorities in AIDS Vaccine Research: One Perspective. *AIDS Research and Human Retroviruses* 8(8): 1431–1432.

Hasskail, H. W. 1981. Legal Problems of Controlled Clinical Trials. *Controlled Clinical Trials* 1: 401–409.

Haynes, B. 1993. Scientific and Social Issues of Human Immunodeficiency Virus Vaccine Development. *Science* 260: 1279–1286.

Heller, P. 1977. Informed Consent and the Old-Fashioned Conscience of the Physician-Investigator. *Perspectives in Biology and Medicine* 20(3): 434–438.

Hellman, S., and Hellman, D. 1991. Of Mice but Not Men: Problems of the Randomized Clinical Trial. *New England Journal of Medicine* 324: 1585–1594.

Helm, A. 1987. Summary of the Presidential Commission for the Study of Ethical Problems and Biomedical and Behavioral Research. *Military Medicine* 152: 425–430.

Helmchen, H. 1981. Problems of Informed Consent in Psychiatry. *Controlled Clinical Trials* 1: 435–440.

Hemminki, E. 1982. Problems of Clinical Trials as Evidence of Therapeutic Effectiveness. *Social Science and Medicine* 16: 711–712.

Henderson, D. 1988. Smallpox and Vaccinia. In *Vaccines*, ed. S. Plotkin and E. Mortimer, pp. 8–30. Philadelphia: W. B. Saunders.

Herman, S. 1989. A Noninstitutional Review Board Comes of Age. *IRB: A Review of Human Subjects Research* 11(2): 1–6.

Hermerén, G. 1983. Human and Social Consequences of Research Ethics. In *Research Ethics*, ed. K. Berg and K. Tranoy, pp. 359–379. New York: Alan Liss, Inc.

Herwaldt, L. 1993. Pertussis and Pertussis Vaccine in Adults. *Journal of the American Medical Association* 269: 53–56.

Hilleman, M. 1975. *Experiments and Research with Humans: Values in Conflict*. Washington, D.C.: National Academy of Science Press.

———. 1985. Newer Directions in Vaccine Development and Utilization. *Journal of*

Infectious Diseases 151(3): 407–419.

——. 1989. An Overview of Technical and Ethical Considerations for the Testing of Experimental AIDS Vaccines in Human Beings, pp. 1–12. Presented at WHO Meeting on Criteria for International Testing and Candidate HIV Vaccines, Geneva, February 27–March 2, 1989.

——. 1992a. Impediments, Imponderables and Alternatives in the Attempt to Develop an Effective Vaccine against AIDS. *Vaccine* 10: 1053–1058.

——. 1992b. The Dilemma of AIDS Vaccines and Therapy: Possible Clues from Comparative Pathogenesis with Measles. *AIDS Research and Human Retroviruses* 8(10): 1743–1748.

Hilleman, M.; Buynak, E.; Roehm, R.; et al. 1975. Purified and Inactivated Human Hepatitis B Vaccine: Progress Report. *American Journal of the Medical Sciences* 270: 401–404.

Hinman, A. 1988. Public Health Considerations. In *Vaccines*, ed. S. Plotkin and E. Mortimer, pp. 587–603. Philadelphia: W. B. Saunders.

Hinman, A.; Bart, K.; and Orenstein, W. 1985. Immunization. In *Infectious Diseases*, 2nd ed., ed. G. Mandell, R. Douglas, and J. Bennett, pp. 1688–1698. New York: John Wiley and Sons.

Hinman, A., and Koplan, J. 1984. Pertussis and Pertussis Vaccine. *Journal of the American Medical Association* 251(23): 3109–3113.

Hoke, C. 1993. Lessons from Field Testing of Non-HIV Vaccines: A Field Trial of Japanese Encephalitis Vaccine in Thailand. *AIDS Research and Human Retroviruses* 9(supp. 1): S161–S167.

Holder, A. 1980. The Case of a Rubella Vaccine Trial. *IRB: A Review of Human Subjects Research* 2(2): 5–7.

Holmes, H. 1989. Can Clinical Research Be Both Ethical and Scientific? *Hypatia* 4(2): 154–165.

Hopps, H.; Meyer, B.; and Parkman, P. 1988. Regulation and Testing of Vaccines. In *Vaccines*, ed. E. Mortimer and S. Plotkin, pp. 576–586. Philadelphia: W. B. Saunders.

Howard, J. 1988. HIV Screening: Scientific, Ethical, and Legal Issues. *Journal of Legal Medicine* 9(4): 601–610.

Howard-Jones, N. 1982. *Human Experimentation and Medical Ethics*. Geneva: World Health Organization.

Huntly, C. 1993. Seeking AIDS Vaccines, Using People in Tests. *Philadelphia Inquirer*, February 8, A1.

Iber, F.; Murray, P.; and Riley, W. A. 1987. *Conducting Clinical Trials*. New York: Plenum Medical Book Co.

Ijsselmuiden, C., and Faden, R. 1992. Research and Informed Consent in Africa: Another Look. *New England Journal of Medicine* 326(12): 830–834.

International Council of Nursing. 1991. Ten Million AIDS Orphans Forecast by Year 2000. *Spotlight: Nursing and HIV/AIDS*, July, 1–2.

IOM/NAS. 1985a. *New Vaccine Development, Establishing Priorities: Diseases of Importance in the United States*. Washington, D.C.: National Academy Press.

——. 1985b. *Vaccine Supply and Innovation*. Washington, D.C.: National Academy Press.

——. 1986. *New Vaccine Development, Establishing Priorities, Volume II: Diseases of Importance in Developing Countries*. Washington, D.C.: National Academy Press.

——. 1988. *Confronting AIDS: Update 1988*. Washington, D.C.: National Academy Press.

——. 1989. *Mobilizing against AIDS*. Cambridge, Mass.: Harvard University Press.

——. 1991. *Expanding Access to Investigational Therapies for HIV and AIDS*. Washington, D.C.: National Academy Press.

Jacobsson, L. 1990. Integrity and Autonomy. In *Ethics in Medicine: Individual In-*

tegrity vs. Demands of Society, ed. P. Allebeck and B. Jansson, pp. 1–21. New York: Raven Press.

Jaffe, H. 1993. Value of Non-vaccine Prevention Research in Trials. *AIDS Research and Human Retroviruses* 9(supp. 1): S151–S152.

Jannson, B. 1990. Ethical Aspects of HIV. In *Ethics in Medicine: Individual Integrity vs. Demands of Society*, ed. P Allebeck and B. Jansson, pp. 179–213. New York: Raven Press.

Jassak, P., and Ryan, M. 1989. Ethical Issues in Clinical Research. *Seminars in Oncology Nursing* 5(2): 102–108.

Jonas, H. 1970. Philosophical Reflections on Experimenting with Human Subjects. In *Experimentation with Human Subjects*, ed. P. Freund, pp. 1–31. New York: George Braziller.

———. 1976. Freedom of Scientific Inquiry and the Public Interest. *Hastings Center Report* 6: 15–17.

Jones, J. 1992. The Tuskegee Legacy: AIDS and the Black Community. *Hastings Center Report* 22(6): 38–40.

Jonsen, A. 1983. A Concord in Medical Ethics. *Annals of Internal Medicine* 99: 261–264.

———. 1989. The Ethics of Using Human Volunteers for High-Risk Research. *Journal of Infectious Diseases* 160(2): 205–208.

———. 1991. Is Individual Responsibility a Sufficient Basis for Public Confidence? *Archives of Internal Medicine* 15(4): 660–662.

Jonsen, A., and Yesley, M. 1980. Rhetoric and Research Ethics: An Answer to Annas. *Medicolegal News* 8(6): 8–13.

Kabat, E. 1975. Ethics and the Wrong Answer. *Science* 189: 505.

Karzon, D.; Bolognesi, D ; and Koff, W. 1992. Development of a Vaccine for the Prevention of AIDS: A Critical Appraisal. *Vaccine* 10(14): 1039–1052.

Katz, J. 1972. *Experimentation with Human Beings*. New York: Russell Sage Foundation.

———. 1974. *Human Rights and Human Experimentation*. Geneva: World Health Organization.

———. 1987. The Regulation of Human Experiments in the U.S.: A Personal Odyssey. *IRB: A Review of Human Subjects Research* 9(1): 1–6.

———. 1992. The Consent Principle of the Nuremberg Code: Its Significance Then and Now. In *The Nazi Doctors and the Nuremberg Code: Human Rights in Human Experimentation*, ed. G. Annas and M. Grodin, pp. 227–239. New York: Oxford University Press.

Katz, J.; Capron, A.; and Glass, E. 1972. Some Basic Questions about Human Research. *Hastings Center Report* 2: 1–2.

Katz, S.; Enders, J.; and Holloway, A. 1960. Studies in Attenuated Measles Virus Vaccine: Clinical, Virologic, and Immunologic Effects of Vaccine in Institutionalized Children. *New England Journal of Medicine* 263(4): 159–161.

Katz, S.; Kempe, H.; Black, F.; Enders, J.; Haggerty, R.; Krugman, S.; and Lepow, M. 1960. Studies of Attenuated Measles Virus Vaccine. *New England Journal of Medicine* 263(4): 180–184.

Katzenstein, D.; Quinnan, G.; and Sawyer, L. 1988. Human Immunodeficiency Virus. In *Vaccines*, ed. S. Plotkin and E. Mortimer, pp. 558–567. Philadelphia: W. B. Saunders Co.

Kaufman, C. 1983. Informed Consent and Patient Decision Making: Two Decades of Research. *Social Science and Medicine* 17(21): 1657–1664.

Kemp, N.; Skinner, E.; and Toms, J. 1984. Randomized Clinical Trials of Cancer Therapy: A Public Opinion Survey. *Clinical Oncology* 10: 155–161.

Kempe, C.; Marsel, J.; Oh, E.; and St. Vincent, L. 1960. Studies in Attenuated Measles Virus Vaccine: Clinical and Antigenic Effects in Institutionalized Children. *New England Journal of Medicine* 263(4): 162–165.

Kessel, E. 1990. Estimated Risks and Benefits in AIDS Vaccine and Drug Trials.

AIDS and Public Policy Journal 5(4): 186–188.

Kessler, D. 1989. The Regulation of Investigational Drugs. *New England Journal of Medicine* 320(5): 281–288.

Keyes, R. 1973. *We, the Lonely People: Searching for Community.* New York: Harper and Row.

Keyserlingk, E. 1990. Ethical Guidelines and Codes: Can They Be Universally Applicable in a Multi-cultural World? In *Ethics in Medicine: Individual Integrity vs. Demands of Society,* ed. P. Allebeck and B. Jansson, pp. 137–149. New York: Raven Press.

Kieffer, G. 1988. Human Experimentation. In *Bio-ethics,* ed. R. Edwards and G. Graber, pp. 196–216. San Diego: Harcourt Brace Jovanovich, Inc.

Kilbourne, E. 1988. Inactivated Influenza Vaccines. In *Vaccines,* ed. S. Plotkin and E. Mortimer, pp. 420–434. Philadelphia: W. B. Saunders.

King, P. 1992. Twenty Years After: The Legacy of the Tuskegee Syphilis Study—The Dangers of Difference. *Hastings Center Report* 22: 35–38.

Kitch, E. 1988. American Law and Preventive Vaccination Programs. In *Vaccines,* ed. S. Plotkin and E. Mortimer, pp. 612–621. Philadelphia: W. B. Saunders.

Kodish, E.; Lantos, J.; and Siegler, M. 1990. Ethical Considerations in Randomized Controlled Clinical Trials. *Cancer* 65(10): 2400–2404.

———. 1991. The Ethics of Randomization. *Cancer* 41(3): 180–186.

Koff, W., and Glass, M. 1992. Future Directions in HIV Vaccine Developments. *AIDS Research and Human Retroviruses* 8(8): 1313–1315.

Koff, W., and Six, H. 1992. *Vaccine Research and Developments.* Vol. I. New York: Marcel Dekker, Inc.

Koff, W.; Wescott, S.; and Hoth, D. 1990. Clinical Trials of AIDS Vaccines. In *AIDS Vaccine Research and Clinical Trials,* ed. S. D. Putney and D. P. Bolognesi, pp. 425–438. New York: Marcel Dekker, Inc.

Kolata, G. 1985. How Safe Are Engineered Organisms? *Science* 229(4708): 34–35.

Koop, C. E. 1988. Individual Freedom and the Public Interest. In *The Global Impact of AIDS,* ed. A. Fleming, M. Carballo, D. FitzSimons, M. Bailey, and J. Mann, pp. 307–311. New York: Alan R. Liss, Inc.

Kopelman, L. 1981. Estimating Risk in Human Research. *Clinical Research* 29: 1–8.

Kostrzewski, J. 1977. Enlisting Community Involvement for Biological Research. *Bulletin of the WHO* 55(supp. 2): 127–132.

Krugman, S. 1983. Further Attenuated Measles Vaccine: Characteristics and Use. *Review of Infectious Diseases* 5: 477–481.

———. 1986. The Willowbrook Hepatitis Studies Revisited: Ethical Aspects. *Review of Infectious Diseases* 8(1): 157–162.

———. 1988. Hepatitis B Vaccine. In *Vaccines,* ed. S. Plotkin and E. Mortimer, pp. 458–473. Philadelphia: W. B. Saunders.

Krugman, S., and Giles, J. 1970. Viral Hepatitis: New Light on an Old Disease. *Journal of the American Medical Association* 212(6): 1019–1029.

Krugman, S.; Giles, J.; and Hammond, J. 1971. Viral Hepatitis, Type B: Studies on Active Immunization. *Journal of the American Medical Association* 217: 41–45.

Krugman, S.; Giles, J.; and Jacobs, A. 1960. Studies of Attenuated Measles Virus Vaccine in Institutionalized Children. *New England Journal of Medicine* 263(4): 174–178.

Kunasol, P. 1993. International HIV/AIDS Vaccine Trials: Expectations of Host Countries. *AIDS Research and Human Retroviruses* 9(supp. 1): S135–S136.

Ladimer, I. 1977. Biological Research for the Community: Legal and Ethical Perspectives. *Bulletin of the WHO* 55(supp. 2): 111–115.

LaMontagne, J., and Curlin, G. 1992. Vaccine Clinical Trials. In *Vaccine Research and Developments,* ed. W. Koff and H. Six, pp. 197–222. New York: Marcel Dekker, Inc.

Lasagna, L. 1980. Regulation and Constraint of Medical Research: Rights and Human Welfare. *Annual Review of Respiratory Diseases* 122: 361–364.

———. 1982. Historical Controls: The Practice of Clinical Trials. *New England Journal of Medicine* 307(21): 1339–1340.

LaVertu, D., and Linares, A. 1990. Ethical Principles of Biomedical Research on Human Subjects, Their Application and Limitations in Latin America and the Caribbean. *Bulletin of PAHO* 24(4): 469–479.

Lebacqz, K. 1977. The National Commission and Research in Pharmacology: An Overview. *Federalism Proceedings* 36(10): 2344–2348.

———. 1980a. Beyond Respect for Persons and Beneficence: Justice in Research. *IRB: A Review of Human Subjects Research* 2(7): 1–4.

———. 1980b. Controlled Clinical Trials: Some Ethical Issues. *Controlled Clinical Trials* 1: 29–36.

Lebacqz, K., and Levine, R. 1977. Respect for Persons and Individual Consent to Participate in Research. *Clinical Research* 25: 101–107.

———. 1979. Ethical Considerations in Clinical Trials. *Clinical Pharmacology and Therapeutics* 25(5): 728–741.

Lecourt, D. 1992. Ethics, Politics, and Medical Obligations in Biomedical Research: The Philosophical Point of View. *AIDS Research and Human Retroviruses* 8: 853–858.

Lehner, T.; Bergneier, L.; and Panagiotidi, L. 1992. Induction of Mucosal and Systemic Immunity to a Recombinant SIV Protein. *Science* 258: 1365–1369.

Lepow, M.; Gray, N.; and Robbins, F. 1960. Studies of Attenuated Measles Virus Vaccine: Clinical, Antigenic, and Prophylactic Effects of Vaccine on Institutionalized and Home-Dwelling Children. *New England Journal of Medicine* 263(4): 170–173.

Levine, C. 1988. Has AIDS Changed the Ethics of Human Subjects Research? *Law, Medicine, and Health Care* 16: 3–4.

———. 1989. *Cases in Bioethics: Selections from Hastings Center Reports*. New York: St. Martin's Press Inc.

———. 1991a. AIDS and the Ethics of Human Subjects Research. In *AIDS and Ethics*, ed. F. Reamer, pp. 77–104. New York: Columbia University Press.

———. 1991b. Children in HIV/AIDS Trials: Still Vulnerable after All These Years. *Law, Medicine, and Health Care* 19(3–4): 231–237.

Levine, C., and Bayer, R. 1989. The Ethics of Screening for Early Intervention of HIV Disease. *American Journal of Public Health* 79(12): 1661–1667.

Levine, C.; Dubler, N.; and Levine, R. 1991. Building a New Consensus: Ethical Principles and Policies for Clinical Research on HIV/AIDS. *IRB: A Review of Human Subjects Research* 13(1–2): 1–17.

Levine, M.; Kaper, J.; Black, R.; and Clements, M. 1983. New Knowledge on the Pathogenesis of Bacterial Enteric Infections as Applied to Vaccine Development. *Microbiology Reviews* 47: 510–550.

Levine, R. 1979. The National Commission Defines the Terms. *Hastings Center Report* 9(3): 21–26.

———. 1982. *Validity of Consent Procedures in Technologically Developing Countries*. Geneva: World Health Organization.

———. 1985. The Use of Placebos in Randomized Clinical Trials. *IRB: A Review of Human Subjects Research* 7(2): 1–4.

———. 1986. *Ethics and Regulation of Clinical Research*. 2nd ed. Baltimore: Urban and Schwarzenberg.

———. 1993. New International Guidelines for Research Involving Human Subjects. *Annals of Internal Medicine* 119(4): 339–341.

Levine, R.; Kanoti, G.; and Lackey, D. 1986. Can a Healthy Subject Volunteer to Be Injured in Research? *Hastings Center Report* 16: 31–33.

Lipsett, M. 1982. On the Nature and Ethics of Phase I Clinical Trials of Cancer Chemotherapy. *Journal of the American Medical Association* 248(8): 941–942.

Lo, B. 1992. Ethical Dilemmas in HIV Infection: What Have We Learned? *Law, Medicine, and Health Care* 20(1–2): 92–103.

Lovell, R. 1990. Ethics, Law, and Resources at the Growing Edge of Medicine. *Australia New Zealand Medicine* 20: 843–849.

Lurie, P.; Bishaw, M.; Chesney, M.; Cooke, M.; Fernandes, M.; Hearst, N.; Katongole-Mbidde, E.; Koetsawang, S.; Lindan, C.; Mandel, J.; Mhloyi, M.; and Coates, T. 1994. Ethical, Behavioral and Social Aspects of HIV Vaccine Trials in Developing Countries. *Journal of the American Medical Association* 271: 295–301.

Lustig, A. 1992. The Method of Principlism: A Critique of the Critique. *Journal of Medicine and Philosophy* 17: 487–510.

Maassab, H.; LaMontagne, J.; and DeBorde, D. 1988. Live Influenza Virus Vaccine. In *Vaccines*, ed. S. Plotkin and E. Mortimer, pp. 435–457. Philadelphia: W. B. Saunders.

Mackillop, W. J., and Johnston, P. A. 1986. Ethical Problems in Clinical Research: The Need for Empirical Studies of the Clinical Trials Process. *Journal of Chronic Diseases* 39(3): 177–188.

Macklin, R. 1977. Consent, Coercion and Conflicts of Rights. *Perspectives in Biology and Medicine* 20: 360–371.

———. 1992. The New Doctors and the Nuremberg Code: Human Rights and Human Experience. In *Universality of the Nuremberg Code*, ed. G. Annas and M. Grodin, pp. 240–257. New York: Oxford University Press.

Macklin, R., and Friedland, G. 1986. AIDS Research: The Ethics of Clinical Trials. *Law, Medicine, and Health Care* 14(5–6): 273–280.

Mahler, H. 1977. Opening Remarks: International Conference on the Role of the Individual and the Community in the Research, Development, and Use of Biologicals. *Bulletin of the WHO* 55(supp. 2): xi.

Maloney, D. 1984. *Protection of Human Research Subjects*. New York: Plenum Press.

Manber, M. 1984. In Search of Medicine's Gold Standard. *Medical World News* 25: 72–92.

Mann, J. 1992. AIDS—The Second Decade: A Global Perspective. *Journal of Infectious Diseases* 165: 245–250.

Mann, J., and Kay, K. 1991. Confronting the Pandemic: The World Health Organization's Global Program on AIDS. *AIDS* 5: S221–S229.

Mann, J.; Tarantola, D.; and Netter, T. (eds.) 1992. *AIDS in the World: The Global AIDS Policy Coalition*. Cambridge, Mass.: Harvard University Press.

Manuel, C.; Enel, P.; Charrel, J.; Reviron, D.; Larher, M.; Thirion, X.; and Sanmarco, J. 1990. The Ethical Approach to AIDS: A Bibliographical Review. *Journal of Medical Ethics* 16: 14–27.

Mariner, W. K. 1989. Why Clinical Trials of AIDS Vaccines Are Premature. *American Journal of Public Health* 79(1): 86–91.

———. 1990. New FDA Drug Approval Policies and HIV Vaccine Development. *American Journal of Public Health* 80(3): 336–341.

———. 1992a. The National Vaccine Injury Compensation Program. *Health Affairs* 11: 255–265.

———. 1992b. AIDS Research and the Nuremberg Code. In *Universality of the Nuremberg Code*, ed. G. Annas and M. Grodin, pp. 286–303. New York: Oxford University Press.

Mariner, W. K., and Gallo, R. C. 1987. Getting to Market: The Scientific and Legal Climate for Developing an AIDS Vaccine. *Law, Medicine, and Health Care* 15: 17–26.

Marini, J.; Sheard, M.; and Bridges, C. 1976. An Evaluation of Informed Consent with Volunteer Prisoner Subjects. *Yale Journal of Biology and Medicine* 49: 427–437.

Marquis, D. 1983. Leaving Treatment to Chance. *Hastings Center Report* 13: 40–47.

Marshall, E. 1986. Does the Moral Philosophy of the Belmont Report Rest on a Mistake? *IRB: A Review of Human Subjects Research* 8: 5–6.

Mathers, P. 1987. Implications of the Federal Drug Investigation and Approval Processes for the Development and Availability of AIDS Treatments and Vaccines. *AIDS Public Policy Journal* 2: 50–53.

Maupas, P.; Goudeau, A.; and Coursaget, P. 1978. Immunization against Hepatitis B in Man: A Pilot Study of Two Years Duration. In *Viral Hepatitis*, ed. G. Vyas, S. Cohen, and R. Schmid, pp. 539–556. Philadelphia: Franklin Institute Press.

Maverick, C. 1979. Hepatitis B Vaccine Trials See Clear Leader in Merck. *American Pharmacy* 19: 132.

McCollum, R.; Randolph, M.; Byrne, E.; and Hilleman, M. 1969. Rubella Virus Vaccine: Antigenic and Protective Efficacy in a Community Trial. *American Journal of Diseases of Children* 118: 186–189.

McCormick, R. 1974. Proxy Consent in the Experimentation Situation. *Perspectives in Biology and Medicine* 18: 2–20.

McIntosh, K.; Cherry, J.; Benenson, A.; Connor, J.; Alling, D.; Rolfe, U.; Todd, W.; Schauberger, J.; and Mattheis, M. 1977. Standard Percutaneous Revaccination of Children Who Received Primary Percutaneous Vaccination. *Journal of Infectious Diseases* 135: 155–165.

Medical Research Council (United Kingdom). 1991. *The Ethical Conduct of AIDS Vaccine Trials. Report of Working Party on Ethical Aspects of AIDS Vaccine Trials.* London: Medical Research Council.

Melton, G.; Levine, R.; Koocher, G.; et al. 1988. Community Consultation in Socially Sensitive Research. *American Psychologist* 43: 573–581.

Merrigan, T. 1990. You Can Teach an Old Dog New Tricks: How AIDS Trials Are Pioneering New Strategies. *New England Journal of Medicine* 323: 1341–1343.

Merz, B. 1988. New Population, New HIV Vaccine in Clinical Trials. *Journal of the American Medical Association* 259: 1290–1291.

Michaels, D., and Levine, C. 1992. Estimates of the Number of Motherless Youth Orphaned by AIDS in the United States. *Journal of the American Medical Association* 268: 3456–3461.

Miller, B. 1987. Experimentation on Human Subjects: The Ethics of Randomized Clinical Trials. In *Health Care Ethics*, ed. D. Vau, D. Veer, and T. Regan, pp. 127–159. Philadelphia: Temple University Press.

Miller, J. 1992. Ethical Standards for Human Subject Research in Developing Countries. *IRB: A Review of Human Subjects Research* 14: 7–8.

Miller, L. 1980. Informed Consent: 1. *Journal of the American Medical Association* 244: 2100.

Miller, S., and Perry, C. 1984. New Lessons Favoring Physicians' Support of Clinical Trials. *American Journal of Medicine* 77: 533–536.

Mitchell, S., and Steingrub, J. 1988. The Changing Clinical Trials Scene: The Role of the IRB. *Institutional Review Board* 10: 1–5.

Mofenson, L.; Wright, P.; and Fast, P. 1992. Summary of the Working Group on Perinatal Intervention. *AIDS Research and Human Retroviruses* 8: 1435–1438.

Morgan, P. 1985. Randomized Clinical Trials Need to Be More Clinical. *Journal of the American Medical Association* 253: 1782–1783.

Mortimer, E. 1988. Pertussis Vaccine. In *Vaccines*, ed. S. Plotkin and E. Mortimer, pp. 74–97. Philadelphia: W. B. Saunders.

Moser, M. 1986. Randomized Clinical Trials: Problems and Values. *American Journal of Emergency Medicine* 4: 173–178.

MRC. *See Medical Research Council*

Murphy, T. 1991. No Time for an AIDS Backlash. *Hastings Center Report* 21: 7–11.

Murray, R. 1969. Biologic Control of Virus Vaccines. *American Journal of Diseases of Children* 118: 334–337.

Muthiah, D.; Kirchkoff, F.; Czajak, S.; Sehgal, P.; and Desrosiers, R. 1992. Protective Effects of a Live Attenuated SIV Vaccine with a Deletion in the NEF Gene. *Science* 258: 1938–1941.

National Commission for the Protection of Human Subjects of Biomedical and Behavioral Research. 1979. *The Belmont Report: Ethical Principles and Guidelines for the Protection of Human Subjects of Research*. Washington, D.C.: U.S. Government Printing Office.

National Commission on Community Health Services. 1966. *Health Is a Community Affair*. Cambridge, Mass.: Harvard University Press.

National Research Council (NRC). 1993. *The Social Impact of AIDS in the United States*. Washington, D.C.: National Academy Press.

Natuk, R.; Chauda, P.; Nubeck, M.; Dans, A.; et al. 1992. Adenovirus–Human Envelope Recombinant Vaccines Elicit Heightened HIV-Neutralizing Antibodies in the Dog Model. *Proceedings of the National Academy of Sciences* 89: 7777–7781.

Naylor, C.; Cher, E.; and Strauss, B. 1992. Measured Enthusiasm: Does the Method of Repeating Trial Results Alter Perceptions of Therapeutic Effectiveness? *Annals of Internal Medicine* 117: 916–921.

Ndinya-Achola, J. 1991. A Review of Ethical Issues in AIDS Research. *East African Medical Journal* 68: 735–740.

Nealon, E.; Blumberg, B.; and Brown, B. 1985. What Do Patients Know about Clinical Trials? *American Journal of Nursing* 85: 807–810.

Nelkin, D. 1983. Public Access vs. Professional Control of Research. In *Research Ethics*, ed. K. Berg and K. Tranoy, pp. 251–258. New York: Alan R. Liss, Inc.

NIAID (National Institute of Allergy and Infectious Diseases). 1991. *Final Report of the Ad Hoc HIV Vaccine Advisory Panel*, July, 1991.

———. 1992. *The Potential Use of HIV Vaccines for the Treatment of HIV Infection: Scientific State of the Art Summary*.

———. 1993a. *Design and Implementation of Vaccine Efficacy Trials*.

———. 1993b. *NIAID Research Agenda for Prophylactic HIV Vaccine Research and Development*.

Nkowane, B.; Wassilak, S.; Orenstein, W.; Bart, K.; Schonberger, L.; Hinman, A.; and Kew, O. 1987. Vaccine Associated Paralytic Poliomyelitis: U.S. 1973–1984. *Journal of the American Medical Association* 257: 1335–1340.

Nokes, K. 1991. Examining the Ethical and Legal Issues Generated by the HIV Epidemic. *Journal of the Association of Nurses in AIDS Care* 2: 25–30.

Novick, A. 1988. Some Ethical Issues Associated with HIV Vaccine Trials. *AIDS Public Policy Journal* 3: 46–48.

———. 1989. Clinical Trials with Vulnerable or Disrespected Subjects. *AIDS Public Policy Journal* 4: 125–130.

Novick, A.; Dubler, N.; and Landesmann, S. 1986. Do Research Subjects Have the Right Not to Know Their HIV Antibody Test Results? *IRB: A Review of Human Subjects Research* 8: 6–9.

NRC. *See National Research Council*

Nzila, N. 1992a. Future Directions. *AIDS Research and Human Retroviruses* 8: 1521–1522.

———. 1992b. Summary of International Trials Working Group. *AIDS Research and Human Retroviruses* 8: 1423–1425.

O'Brien, M. 1979. Legal Implications of the Use of Vaccines. *Medico-Legal Journal* 47: 152–159.

Osborn, J. 1978. In the Matter of Witch Hunts. *Journal of the American Medical*

Association 240: 1616–1617.

Oseasohn, R. 1988. Cholera. In *Vaccines*, ed. S. Plotkin and E. Mortimer, pp. 362–371. Philadelphia: W. B. Saunders.

Panem, S. 1985. AIDS: Public Policy and Biomedical Research. *Hastings Center Report* 15: 23–26.

Pantaleo, G.; Graziosi, C.; Demarest, J.; Butini, L.; Montroni, M.; Fox, C.; Orenstein, J.; Kotler, D.; and Fauci, A. 1993. HIV Infection Is Active and Progressive in Lymphoid Tissue during the Clinically Latent Stage of Disease. *Nature* 362: 355–358.

Pape, J.; Deschaveys, M.; Verdier, R.; et al. 1992. The Urge for an AIDS Vaccine: Perspectives from a Developing Country. *AIDS Research and Human Retroviruses* 8: 1535–1537.

Pappworth, M. H. 1967. *Human Guinea Pigs: Experimentation on Man*. London: Routledge and Kegan Paul.

Parish, H. J. 1968. *Victory with Vaccines*. Edinburgh and London: E. and S. Livingstone Ltd.

Peckman, P. 1983. Informed Consent: Ethical, Legal and Medical Implications. *British Medical Journal* 286: 1117–1121.

Pellegrino, E. 1990a. Ethics. *Journal of the American Medical Association* 263: 2641–2642.

———. 1990b. The Relationship of Autonomy and Integrity in Medical Ethics. In *Bioethics Issues and Perspectives*, ed. S. Connor and H. Fuenzalida-Puelma, pp. 8–17. Washington, D.C.: PAHO.

———. 1993. The Metamorphosis of Medical Ethics. *Journal of the American Medical Association* 269; 1158–1162.

Peter, G. 1985. Vaccine Crisis: An Emerging Societal Problem. *Journal of Infectious Diseases* 151: 981–983.

Peterman, T., and Sevgi, A. 1993. Evaluating Behavioral Interventions: Need for Randomized Controlled Trials. *Journal of the American Medical Association* 269: 2845.

Petricciani, J.; Gracher, V.; Sizaret, A.; and Regan, P. 1989. Vaccines: Obstacles and Opportunities from Discovery to Use. *Review of Infectious Diseases* 11: S524–S529.

Petricciani, J.; Koff, W.; and Ada, G. 1992. Efficacy Trials for HIV/AIDS Vaccines. *AIDS Research and Human Retroviruses* 8: 1527–1529.

Pichichero, M. E.; Green, J. L.; Francis, A. B.; Marsocci, S. M.; and Disney, F. A. 1990. New Vaccines and Vaccination Policies. *Pediatric Annals* 19(12): 686–694.

Pietroban, P., and Kauda, P. 1992. Lysopeptides and Their Effects on the Immune System. In *Vaccine Research and Development*, vol. 1, ed. W. Koff and H. Six, pp. 3–29. New York: Marcel Dekker, Inc.

Plotkin, S. 1988. Rubella Vaccine. In *Vaccines*, ed. S. Plotkin and E. Mortimer, pp. 235–262. Philadelphia: W. B. Saunders.

Plotkin, S.; Cornfeld, D.; and Ingalls, T. 1965. Studies of Immunization with Lung Rubella Virus: Trials in Children with a Strain Cultured from an Aborted Fetus. *American Journal of Diseases of Children* 110: 381–389.

Plotkin, S.; Farquhar, J.; Katz, M.; and Buser, F. 1969. Attentuation of RA 27/3 Rubella Virus in WI-38 Human Diploid Cells. *American Journal of Diseases of Children* 118: 301.

Plotkin, S.; Ingalls, T.; and Farquhar, J. 1968. Intranasally Administered Rubella Vaccine. *Lancet* 2: 934.

Plotkin, S., and Mortimer, E. (eds.). 1988. *Vaccines*. Philadelphia: W. B. Saunders.

Plotkin, S., and Plotkin, S. 1985. Vaccination: One Hundred Years Later. In *World's Debt to Pasteur: Proceedings of a Centennial Symposium Commemorating the First Rabies Vaccine*, ed. H. Koprowski and S. Plotkin, pp. 83–106. New York:

Alan Liss.

———. 1988. A Short History of Vaccination. In *Vaccines*, ed. S. Plotkin and E. Mortimer, pp. 1–7. Philadelphia: W. B. Saunders.

Porter, J.; Glass, M.; and Koff, W. 1989. Ethical Considerations in AIDS Vaccine Testing. *IRB: A Review of Human Subjects Research* 11(3): 1–4.

Porterfield, J. 1988. Aberrant Responses to Infectious Agents: Immune Enhancement of Viral Infectivity. In *Technological Advances in Vaccine Development: Proceedings of a Genentech, Ortho, Smith Kline and French–UCLA Symposium*, ed. L. Lasky, pp. 539–546. New York: Alan Liss, Inc.

Preblud, S., and Katz, S. 1988. Measles Vaccine. In *Vaccines*, ed. S. Plotkin and E. Mortimer, pp. 182–222. Philadelphia: W. B. Saunders.

President's Commission for the Study of Ethical Problems in Medicine and in Biomedical and Behavioral Research. 1982. *Compensating for Research Injuries*. Washington, D.C.: Government Printing Office.

Price, M. 1989. *Shattered Mirrors: Our Search for Identity and Community in the AIDS Era*. Cambridge, Mass.: Harvard University Press.

Priester, R. 1992. A Values Framework for Health System Reform. *Health Affairs* 11: 84–107.

Purcell, R., and Gerin, J. 1978. Hepatitis B Vaccines: A Status Report. In *Viral Hepatitis*, ed. G. Vyas, S. Cohen, and R. Schmid, pp. 491–505. Philadelphia: Franklin Institute Press.

Rawlins, M. 1989. Trading Risk for Benefit. In *Risk and Consent to Risk in Medicine*, ed. R. Mann, pp. 193–202. Park Ridge, N.J.: Parthenon Publishing Group.

Reamer, F. 1991. AIDS: The Relevance of Ethics. In *AIDS and Ethics*, ed. F. Reamer, pp. 1–25. New York: Columbia University Press.

1991. *Research Issues in Human Behavior and Sexually Transmitted Diseases in the AIDS Era*. Washington, D.C.: American Society for Microbiology.

Richman, D. 1989. Public Access to Experimental Drug Therapy: AIDS Raises Yet Another Conflict between Freedom of the Individual and Welfare of the Individual and Public. *Journal of Infectious Diseases* 159(3): 412–415.

Rida, W.; Meier, P.; and Stevens, C. 1993. Design and Implementation of Efficacy Trials. *AIDS Research and Human Retroviruses* (supp. 1): S59–S64.

Riddinough, M.; Sisk, J.; and Bell, J. 1983. Influenza Vaccination: Cost Effectiveness and Public Policy. *Journal of the American Medical Association* 249: 3189–3195.

Riis, P. 1990. Clinical Freedom: Patients and Physicians' Autonomy versus the Demands of Society. In *Ethics in Medicine*, ed. P. Allebeck and B. Jannson, pp. 103–113. New York: Raven Press.

Robbins, A., and Freeman, P. 1988. Obstacles to Developing Vaccines for the Third World. *Scientific American* 259: 126–133.

Robbins, F. 1977. The Demand for Human Trials in Biological Research. *Bulletin of the WHO* 55: 73–84.

———. 1979. Criteria of Informed Consent in Vaccine Trials. In *Human Experimentation and the Protection of Human Rights*, ed. N. Howard-Jones and Z. Bankowski, pp. 211–217. Geneva: CIOMS.

———. 1986. AIDS: A Classical Public Health Problem in Modern Guise. In *AIDS: Impact on Public Policy*, ed. R. Hummel, W. Leavy, M. Rampolla, and S. Charost. New York: Plenum Press.

———. 1988. Polio—Historical. In *Vaccines*, ed. S. Plotkin and E. Mortimer, pp. 98–114. Philadelphia: W. B. Saunders.

Roberts, C. 1982. Biology and the New Age: An Evolutionary and Ethical Assessment. *Perspectives in Biology and Medicine* 25: 176–193.

Rodwin, M. 1989. Preventing AIDS: Self-interest and Public Spirit. *AIDS Public Policy Journal* 4: 120.

Roginsky, M. 1982. Clinical Trials of New Drugs: Special Problems. In *Human Subjects: A Handbook for IRBs*, ed. R. Greenwald, M. Ryan, and J. Mulinhill, pp. 181–192. New York: Plenum Press.

Rosner, F. 1987. The Ethics of Randomized Controlled Trials. *American Journal of Medicine* 82: 283–290.

Rosser, S. 1989. Re-visioning Clinical Research: Gender and the Ethics of Experimental Design. *Hypatia* 4: 127–139.

Rothman, D. 1987a. Ethics and Human Experimentation: Henry Beecher Revisited. *New England Journal of Medicine* 317: 1195–1199.

———. 1987b. Ethical and Social Issues in the Development of New Drugs and Vaccines. *Bulletin of the New York Academy of Medicine* 63(6): 557–568.

Rothman, D., and Edgar, H. 1991. AIDS, Activism, and Ethics. *Hospital Practice* 26: 135–142.

———. 1992. Scientific Rigor and Medical Realities: Placebo Trials in Cancer and AIDS Research. In *AIDS: The Making of a Chronic Disease*, ed. E. Fee and D. Fox, pp. 194–206. Berkeley: University of California Press.

Sabin, A. 1985. Oral Poliovirus Vaccine: History of Its Development and Age and Current Challenge to Eliminate Poliomyelitis from the World. *Journal of Infectious Diseases* 151: 420–436.

———. 1992. Improbability of Effective Vaccination against HIV Because of Its Intracellular Transmission and Rectal Portal of Entry. *Proceedings of the National Academy of Sciences* 89: 8852–8855.

Sachs, L. 1990. Integrity and Autonomy from an Anthropological Point of View. In *Ethics in Medicine*, ed. P. Allebeck and B. Jannson, pp. 33–46. New York: Raven Press.

Sacks, H.; Chalmers, T.; and Smith, H. 1982. Randomized vs. Historical Controls for Clinical Trials. *American Journal of Medicine* 72: 233–240.

Salk, J. 1987. Prospects for the Control of AIDS by Immunizing Seropositive Individuals. *Nature* 327: 473–476.

Sass, H.-M. 1990. Bioethics: Its Philosophical Basis and Application. In *Bioethics: Issues and Perspectives*, ed. S. Connor and H. Fuenzalida-Puelma, pp. 18–23. Washington, D.C.: PAHO.

———. 1992. Introduction: The Principle of Solidarity in Health Care Policy. *Journal of Medicine and Philosophy* 17: 367–370.

Sawyer, L.; Katzenstein, D.; and Quinnan, G. 1988. Regulatory Concerns regarding AIDS Vaccine Development. *AIDS Public Policy Journal* 3: 36–45.

Schafer, A. 1982. The Ethics of the Randomized Clinical Trial. *New England Journal of Medicine* 307: 719–724.

———. 1985. The Randomized Controlled Trial: For Whose Benefit? *IRB: A Review of Human Subjects Research* 7: 4–6.

Schiff, G.; Donath, R.; and Rotte, T. 1969. Experimental Rubella Studies: Clinical and Laboratory Features of Infection Caused by Rubella Virus—Artificial Challenge Studies of Adult Rubella Vaccines. *American Journal of Diseases of Children* 118: 269–276.

Schild, G. C., and Minor, P. D. 1990. Modern Vaccines: Human Immunodeficiency Virus and AIDS—Challenges and Progress. *Lancet* 335: 1081–1084.

Schipper, H. 1985. Why Are Patients Not Entered into Clinical Trials? *Cancer Investigation* 3: 97–98.

Schooley, R. 1988. The Quest for an AIDS Vaccine. *New England Journal of Public Policy* 4: 135–144.

Schultz, A., and Hu, S. 1993. Primate Models for HIV Vaccines. *AIDS* 7(supp. 1): S161–S170.

Schumacher, W. 1979. Legal/Ethical Aspects of Vaccinations. *Developments in Biological Standardization* 43: 435–438.

Schwartz, D.; Gorse, G.; Clements, M.; Belshe, R.; Izu, A.; Duliege, A.; Berman, P.;

Twaddell, T.; Stablein, D.; Sposto, R.; Siliciano, R.; and Matthews, T. 1993. Induction of HIV-1 Neutralising and Syncytium-Inhibiting Antibodies in Uninfected Recipients of HIV-1(IIIB) rgp120 Subunit Vaccine. *Lancet* 342: 69–73.

Scolnick, E.; McLean, A.; West, D.; McAleer, W.; Miller, W.; and Buynak, E. 1984. Clinical Evaluation in Healthy Adults of a Hepatitis B Vaccine Made by Recombinant DNA. *Journal of the American Medical Association* 251: 2812–2815.

Selik, R.; Chu, S.; and Buehler, J. 1993. HIV Infection as Leading Cause of Death among Young Adults in U.S. Cities and States. *Journal of the American Medical Association* 269: 2991–2994.

Shorr, A. 1992. AIDS and the FDA: An Ethical Case for Limiting Patient Access to New Medical Therapies. *IRB: A Review of Human Subjects Research* 14: 1–5.

Silverman, W. 1989. The Myth of IC: In Daily Practice and in Clinical Trials. *Journal of Medical Ethics* 15: 6–11.

Smith, L., and Brennan, R. 1987. Legal Ramifications of the Development of an AIDS Vaccine. *New England Journal of Medicine* 84: 702–705.

Smith, P.; Hayes, R.; and Mulder, D. 1991. Epidemiological and Public Health Considerations in the Design of HIV Vaccine Trials. *AIDS* 5: S105–S111.

Smith, P., and Morrow, R. 1991. *Methods for Field Trials of Interventions against Tropical Diseases: A Toolbox*. New York: Oxford University Press.

Snow, W. 1992. International Conference on Advances in AIDS Vaccine Development. *AIDS Research and Human Retroviruses* 8: 1433–1434.

———. 1993. Efficacy Trials, Design and Implementation: Working with the Community. *AIDS Research and Human Retroviruses* 9(supp. 1): S153–S154.

Spicker, S.; Alon, I.; de Vries, A.; and Engelhardt, H. T. 1988. *The Use of Human Beings in Research*. Dordrecht: Kluwer Academic Publishers.

Spodick, D. 1982. The Controlled Clinical Trial: Medicine's Most Powerful Tool. *Humanist* 42: 12–21.

Stein, R. 1992. The Development of an HIV Vaccine. In *Vaccine Research and Clinical Trials*, ed. W. Koff and H. Six, pp. 223–244. New York: Marcel Dekker, Inc.

Stein, R., and Jessop, D. 1983. An Ethics Committee to Aid in Implementing a Randomized Clinical Trial. *Controlled Clinical Trials* 4: 37–42.

Stevens, C.; Taylor, P.; Tong, M.; Toy, P.; Vyas, G.; Nair, P.; et al. 1987. Yeast-Recombinant HB Vaccine: Efficacy with Hepatitis B Immune Globulin in Prevention of Perinatal Hepatitis B Virus Transmission. *Journal of the American Medical Association* 257: 2612–2616.

Stolley, P. 1993. The Hazards of Misguided Compassion. *Annals of Internal Medicine* 118: 822–823.

Stuart-Harris, C. 1980. The Present Status of Live Influenza Virus Vaccine. *Journal of Infectious Diseases* 142: 784–792.

Sullivan, L. 1991. Partners in Prevention: A Mobilization Plan for Implementing Healthy People 2000. *American Journal of Health Promotion* 5: 291–297.

Sundstrom, P. 1991. AIDS, Myths and Ethics. *Theoretical Medicine* 12: 151–156.

Szmuness, W.; Stevens, C.; Harley, E.; Zang, E.; Oleszko, W.; William, D.; Sadovsky, R.; Morrison, J.; and Kellner, A. 1980. Hepatitis B Vaccine: Demonstration of Efficacy in a Controlled Clinical Trial in a High Risk Population in the United States. *New England Journal of Medicine* 303: 833–841.

Tacket, C., and Edelman, R. 1991. Ethical Issues Involving Volunteers in AIDS Vaccine Trials. *Journal of Infectious Diseases* 161(2): 356.

Tancredi, L. 1975. The Ethics Quagmire and Random Clinical Trials. *Inquiry* 12(3): 171–179.

Tarantola, D. 1988. Global Strategy for the Prevention and Control of AIDS. In *The Global Impact of AIDS*, ed. A. Fleming, M. Carballo, D. FitzSimons, M. Bailey, and J. Mann, pp. 207–214. New York: Alan R. Liss, Inc.

Taylor, K., and Kelner, M. 1987. Informed Consent: The Physician's Perspective. *Social Science and Medicine* 24: 135–143.

Taylor, K.; Mayolese, R.; and Soskolne, C. 1984. Physician's Reasons for Not Entering Eligible Patients in a Randomized Clinical Trial of Surgery for Breast Cancer. *New England Journal of Medicine* 310: 1363–1367.

Thomas, S., and Quinn, S. 1991. The Tuskegee Syphilis Study: Implications for HIV Education and AIDS Risk Education Programs in the Black Community. *American Journal of Public Health* 81: 1498–1504.

Thomasma, D. 1983. Beyond Medical Paternalism and Patient Autonomy: A Model of Physician Convenience. *Annals of Internal Medicine* 98: 243–248.

Thong, Y. H., and Harth, S. C. 1991. The Social Filter Effect of Informed Consent in Clinical Research. *Pediatrics* 87(4): 568–569.

Toomey, K.; Cahill, K.; et al. 1988. Partner Notification. *New England Journal of Medicine* 319: 442.

Toulmin, S. 1981. The Tyranny of Principles. *Hastings Center Report* 11: 31–39.

Tranoy, K. E. 1990. The Roots of Medical Ethics in a Shared Morality. In *Ethics in Medicine*, ed. P. Allebeck and B. Jannson, pp. 23–31. New York: Raven Press.

Twomey, J. 1989. The Ethics of Clinical Research with Children with HIV Infection. *Virginia Nurse* 57: 38–43.

Tydskuf, S. A. 1977. When Is Experience with History Inadmissible? *Afrikaans* 52: 342.

Uberla, K. 1981. Randomized Clinical Trials: Why Not? *Controlled Clinical Trials* 1: 295–303.

U.S. Department of Health and Human Services. 1992. *NIH Data Book 1992*. Bethesda, Md.: NIH.

U.S. Public Health Service (USPHS). 1988. Report of the Second Public Health Service AIDS Prevention and Control Conference. *Public Health Report* 103(supp. 1): 1–98.

———. 1991. U.S. Public Health Service Consultation on International Collaborative Human Immunodeficiency Virus Research. *Law, Medicine, and Health Care* 19: 259–263.

Vaheri, A.; Vesikari, T.; Oker-Blon, N.; Seppala, M.; Veronelli, J.; Robbins, F.; and Parkman, P. 1969. Transmission of Attenuated Rubella Vaccines to the Human Fetus. *American Journal of Diseases of Children* 118: 243–251.

Veatch, R. 1983. Justice and Research Design: The Case of the Semi-randomized Clinical Trial. *Clinical Research* 31: 12–22.

———. 1987. *The Patient as Partner: A Theory of Human Experimentation Ethics*. Bloomington and Indianapolis: Indiana University Press.

Vere, D. W. 1978. Selection and Recruitment of Healthy Subjects in Research. In *Medical Experimentation and the Protection of Human Rights*, ed. N. Howard-Jones and Z. Bankowski. Geneva: CIOMS/WHO.

———. 1981. Controlled Clinical Trial: The Current Ethical Debate. *Journal of the Royal Society of Medicine* 74: 85–88.

———. 1983. Problems in Controlled Trials: A Critical Response. *Journal of Medical Ethics* 9: 85–89.

Vermund, S. 1994. The Efficacy of Human Immunodeficiency Virus Vaccines: Methodological Issues in Preparing for Clinical Trials. In *Models and Methods of Epidemiologic Research on HIV Infection*, ed. A. Nicolosi, pp. 1–21. New York: Raven Press.

Vermund, S.; Fischer, R.; Hoff, R.; Rida, W.; Sheon, A.; Lawrence, D.; Hoth, D.; and Barker, L. 1993. Preparing for HIV Vaccine Efficacy Trials: Partnerships and Challenges. *AIDS Research and Human Retroviruses* 9(supp. 1): S127–S132.

Vermund, S.; Hoff, R.; Lawrence, D.; Fischer, R.; Reda, W.; Fast, P.; Koff, W.; Ungar, B.; Hoth, D.; and Barker, L. 1992. HIV Vaccine Efficacy Trial Preparations.

VIII International Conference on AIDS (Abstract). POC 4505

Volberding, P., and Abrams, D. 1985. Clinical Care and Research in AIDS. *Hastings Center Report* 15: 16–18.

Waldenstein, J. 1983. The Ethics of Randomization. In *Research Ethics*, ed. K. Berg and K. Tranoy, pp. 243–249. New York: Alan R. Liss, Inc.

Walters, L. 1988. Ethical Issues in the Prevention and Treatment of HIV Infection and AIDS. *Science* 239: 597–603.

Weintraub, M. 1983. Improving the Ethics of Clinical Trials: The Case of an Add-on Study. *IRB: A Review of Human Subjects Research* 5: 7–8.

Weisburd, S. 1987. AIDS Vaccines: The Problem of Human Testing. *Science News* 131: 329–332.

Weisse, A. 1991. *Medical Odysseys*. New Brunswick, N.J.: Rutgers University Press.

Westrin, C.; Nilstun, T.; Smedby, B.; and Haglund, B. 1992. Epidemiology and Moral Philosophy. *Journal of Medical Ethics* 18: 193–196.

WHO/GPA. 192. *Second Meeting on AIDS Drug and Vaccine Supply*. Geneva: WHO.

Wiktor, T.; Plotkin, S.; and Koprowski, H. 1988. Rabies Vaccine. In *Vaccines*, ed. S. Plotkin and E. Mortimer, pp. 474–491. Philadelphia: W. B. Saunders.

Wilhelmsen, L. 1979. Ethics of Clinical Trials: The Use of Placebo. *European Journal of Clinical Pharmacology* 16: 295–297.

Wilkins, J.; Leedom, J.; Portnoy, B.; and Salvatore, M. 1969. Reinfection with Rubella Virus Despite Live Vaccine Induced Immunity. *American Journal of Diseases of Children* 118: 275–294.

Williams, G. 1959. *Virus Hunters*. New York: Alfred A. Knopf.

Wittek, A., and Quinnan, G. 1990. AIDS Vaccines: Regulatory, Scientific and Ethical Issues. In *AIDS Vaccine Research and Clinical Trials*, ed. S. Putney and S. Bolognesi, pp. 439–469. New York: Marcel Dekker, Inc.

Woodward, W.; Gilman, R.; Horvick, R.; Libonati, J.; and Cash, R. 1976. Efficacy of a Live Oral Cholera Vaccine in Human Volunteers. *Developments in Biological Standardization* 33: 108–112.

World Health Organization. *See WHO/GPA*

Wyatt, H. V. 1973. Is Polio a Model for Consumer Research? *Nature* 241: 247–249.

———. 1977. Vaccines and Social Responsibility: Here Are Some Answers, What Are the Questions? *Moralist* 60: 81–95.

Young, F.; Norris, J.; Levitt, J.; and Nightingale, S. 1988. The FDA's New Procedure for the Use of Investigational Drugs in Treatment. *Journal of the American Medical Association* 259: 2267–2270.

Zagury, D.; Leonard, R.; Fouchard, M.; Reveil, B.; Bernard, J.; Ittele, D.; Cattone, A.; Zirimbuabagabo, L.; Kalumbo, M.; Justin, W.; Salaon, J.; and Goussard, B. 1987. Immunization against AIDS in Humans. *Nature* 326: 249–250.

Zelen, M. 1982. Strategy and Alternate Randomized Designs in Cancer Clinical Trials. *Cancer Treatment Reports* 66: 1095–1100.

Zuckerman, A. 1986. Why Vaccines? *Journal of Infection* 13: 1.

Zuckerman, A. J. 1988. The Enigma of AIDS Vaccines. In *The Global Impact of AIDS*, ed. A. Fleming, M. Carballo, D. FitzSimons, M. Bailey, and J. Mann, pp. 375–384. New York: Alan R. Liss.

Index

▼

47, 61; Global Programme on AIDS and network for isolation and characterization of HIV subtypes, 100; infrastructure development for HIV vaccine efficacy trials, 113; transfer of patent rights for antimalaria vaccine to, 160n.50

World Medical Association, 39, 61. *See also* Declaration of Helsinki

World War II, human-subjects research during, 34–35, 58

Yellow fever, history of vaccination, 16

Zagury, Dr. Daniel, 101–102

Zaire, clinical testing of HIV vaccine in, 102, 123

Zidovudine (AZT), 2, 50, 161n.54

Christine Grady is Acting Clinical Director and Research Associate at the National Institute of Nursing Research, the National Institutes of Health. She has served as a member of the staff of the President's Commission on the HIV Epidemic and has been involved in the care of patients with HIV and research in the area of HIV infection since 1983.

137
140